THE LONGEVITY
STRATEGY

THE LONGEVITY STRATEGY

How to Live to 100 Using the Brain-Body Connection

DAVID MAHONEY
RICHARD RESTAK

FOREWORD BY WILLIAM SAFIRE

THE
DANA
PRESS

John Wiley & Sons, Inc.

New York • Chichester • Weinheim • Brisbane • Singapore • Toronto

Copyright © 1998 by David Mahoney and Richard Restak.
All rights reserved

Published by John Wiley & Sons, Inc.
Published simultaneously in Canada
Design and production by Navta Associates, Inc.

This publication is designed to provide accurate and authoritative information in regard to the subject matter covered. It is sold with the understanding that the publisher is not engaged in rendering professional services. If professional advice or other expert assistance is required, the services of a competent professional person should be sought.

Library of Congress Cataloging-in-Publication Data:
Mahoney, David J.
 The longevity strategy : how to live to 100 using the brain-body
 connection / David Mahoney, Richard Restak.
  p. cm.
 Includes index.
 ISBN 0-471-24867-3 (cloth : alk. paper)
  1. Longevity. 2. Mind and body. Brain—Aging.
I. Restak, Richard M., 1942– . II. Title.
RA776.75.M1156 1998
613—dc21   97-50639
                                                                CIP

Printed in the United States of America

10 9 8 7 6 5 4 3 2

CONTENTS

ACKNOWLEDGMENTS

David Mahoney—No one is who he is without family support. So acknowledgment is due to my three supportive sons and their loving wives who have given me six spectacular grandchildren. Their futures are the purpose of this book.

To William Safire—a figurative "brother" for almost forty years—my respect, affection, and appreciation. He lives and defines the meaning of loyalty and friendship.

Due to the subject, most people listed are from the medical or scientific fields. Yet many nonscientists—friends, teachers, coaches, and teammates—have shared in my ongoing longevity. It is impossible to acknowledge each friend or associate who has directly or indirectly contributed to this work, but I want to try: Cary Akins, Marilyn Albert, Robert Barchi, Kenneth Beer, Baruj Benacerraf, Colin Blakemore, Floyd Bloom, Nancy Brinker, William Cahan, Edwin Cassem, Francis Collins, Leon Cooper, W. Maxwell Cowan, Joseph Coyle; the Charles A. Dana Foundation Board of Directors (Edward C. Andrews Jr., Wallace L. Cook, Walter G. Corcoran, Charles A. Dana Jr., Donald B. Marron, Ann McLaughlin, Carlos Moseley, L. Guy Palmer II, Edward F. Rover, William L. Safire, Herbert Siegel, and Clark M. Whittemore Jr.), the Eleanor Naylor Dana Trustees (Robert A. Good, Carlos Moseley, A. J. Signorile, and Robert E. Wise), Horace Deets, Roman DeSanctis, Angie Dickinson, Roy Duke, Gerald Fischbach, Marjorie Fisher, Anne Sutherland Fuchs, Barbara Gill, Murray Goldstein, Enoch Gordis, Vartan Gregorian, Zach Hall, Joseph Hayes, Bernadine Healy, Henry Heimlich, Norbert Herschkowitz, Don Hewitt, Steven E. Hyman, Kay Jamison, Lauren Kearns, Istvan Krisko, LaSalle Leffall, Alan Leshner, the Hon. John Lindsay, Pierre Magistretti, Robert and

Helene Mahoney, Patricia Mangini, Christian Marich, Joseph Martin, Douglas Mathisen, Guy McKhann, Grace Mirabella, Daniel J. Moriarty, David Nathan, Jane Nevins, James Nicholas, Pascal Nicod, Gerald O'Connor, Herbert Pardes, Michael Phelps, Warren Phillips, Fred Plum, Stanley Prusiner, Stuart Quan, the Hon. Paul Rogers, Bruce Rosen, Edward Rover, Lewis Rowland, Pete Rozelle, Carla Shatz, Herbert Siegel, Irwin Smigel, the Hon. Ted Stevens, Piergiorgio Strata, Suzanne Sunshine, Samuel Thier, Daniel Tosteson, Garrick Utley, Mike Wallace, Donald Warren, James Watson, and Ernst Wynder. My gratitude to each, and my apologies to those I may have unconsciously omitted. I am grateful to all who have been a part of my life.

My thanks also to the foundation staff, which, in many ways, I feel is our greatest accomplishment. We have recruited and trained some of the finest young executives I have ever met. That says a lot.

No acknowledgment could be complete without expressing my thanks to Richard Restak. He is both a professional and a friend, and I value our relationship.

Richard Restak—In addition to many of the above, my special thanks to the following for suggestions, interviews, discussions, and helpful criticism: Linda Bruce, Art Buchwald, Robert Butler, Carl Cotman, Donna de Varona, Stanley Jacobson, S. Michal Jazwinski, Leonard Poon, Michael Scheier, Burton S. Singer, and Wayne M. Sotile. Our great appreciation also to Randy Talley of the Dana Press and the editorial team at Wiley: Gerry Helferich, Carole Hall, Tom Miller, and John Simko. Very special thanks to William Safire for reading the early version of our manuscript and making many helpful suggestions. Finally, my thanks to David Mahoney, whose courtesy, wit, and focus made the process of coauthorship such a delight.

FOREWORD

THE SCENE WAS A BLACK-TIE dinner at the Swedish Embassy in Washington, D.C. The host was Rolf Ekeus, who had led the U.N. commission searching for Saddam Hussein's biological warfare sites and was the new Swedish ambassador. The guests of honor were five American scientists who won Nobel prizes in 1997.

I posed this question to the Nobel laureates: If Albert Einstein were a young man just starting his career today, what field would he choose to work in?

"Einstein was not only a genius, he was a smart guy," replied one of the scientists. "I think he would choose a field of science with the greatest potential for dramatic advances in his lifetime, as he did at the start of the twentieth century by choosing physics."

"Which field would that be today?"

"Molecular biology."

"Ah," said a voice from one of the tables, "neuroscience. The brain."

Even the physicists and chemists and doctors in the room—pioneers in their chosen disciplines of some of the most exciting advances of our time—had to agree.

Let's assume these guys are right. It may well be that discoveries in brain science—propelled by techniques of imaging that let us see thinking in action, and by feats of genetic engineering and chemical therapy—will lead to breakthroughs that will unleash the power of the brain to better control the workings of the body.

What does this assumption mean to thee and me? First, it means that new hope and purpose are given to the growing likelihood of longevity. We already know that the lives of human beings are stretching out, and the speed of the stretching and of the typical life span is likely to accelerate. Thanks to antibiotics and other advances in medical science, you are expected to live about ten years longer than your great-grandfather. And thanks to organ transplants and gene therapy, as well as the strong likelihood of cures for cancer and protections against heart disease and stroke, your grandchildren are expected to live more than a decade longer than you. Since life expectancy has risen from forty-seven to seventy-five in the twentieth century, isn't it likely to rise to 100 in the twenty-first?

Too many people in politics and medicine think of this as a terrible problem. They wonder—what are we going to do with all those old people? How will we manage the burden of an aging population?

Others are thinking more positively. These more upbeat futurists wonder—what can brain science do to keep the mind active, alert, and productive into the years that used to be reserved for rocking chairs and nursing homes? What can people do for themselves, right now, to prepare themselves for—indeed to take advantage of—the longer life that the scientists of brain and body are making possible?

That's what this book by David Mahoney and Richard Restak is about. I wasn't born yesterday (actually, I was born sixty-eight years ago) and I'm not kidding myself; even with all the cures in the pipeline, and even if I buckle my seat belt all the time, the odds are against my living to 100. But I'm *planning* to live to 100. How can this be? Are not those two statements inconsistent?

Not a bit. According to Mahoney and Restak, the way to take advantage of the growing opportunity most of us have to live longer, and then to pack enjoyment and fulfillment into that extended life, is to adopt a strategy of longevity.

"Strategy" can be one of those con-job words. In this case, however—as I get it from reading this book and from a lifetime of working with David—the longevity strategy is to act along the range of our personal fronts, over a period of the rest of our lives, in a way that will make our fourth quarter the lively culmination of the first three. This takes specific planning for physical health, for mental acuity, for financial security, for family and friendships, and for the systematic shifts in emphasis of career and avocation that keep the mind alert and spirit alive.

The bonus to their longevity strategy, say the authors, is this: in our first three generations of life, we benefit from the security and perspective that comes with knowing roughly what we're preparing for our fourth—"the last of life, for which the first was made." Precisely because we are determined not to vegetate as grumpy codgers, and because we take full advantage of what's being learned about brain-body interaction, we are more likely to be happily productive pre-geezers.

The authors have the credentials to be longevity strategists. They know they're not likely to get a "Happy Hundredth Birthday!" waved at them from a wrinkled Willard Scott on some far-off day, but they combine the experience needed to put together their wide-ranging plan. One is a marketing genius turned activist-philanthropist, the other a medical doctor who also practices understandable writing in best-seller form.

Let me tell you about David; how he involved me in the publicizing of brain science; what makes him so important to so many neuroscientists; and why I egged him on when he came up with the idea for writing this book.

The Nobel laureate James Watson, co-discoverer of DNA a generation ago and today the father of the international Human Genome Project, will be remembered as one of the half dozen scientists who—like Einstein—most moved human knowledge forward in the twentieth century. With all his prestige, and with his reputation for being an outspoken coot who doesn't stand on ceremony, he was able to assemble some of the leading lights in his field at his laboratory in Cold Spring Harbor, Long Island, to listen to a challenge from a non-scientist.

David had started his career working in the mail room of an ad agency while taking night classes at the University of Pennsylvania. He rode his marketing genius to the top of one of America's largest consumer companies and then started a second career as a philanthropist, ultimately becoming CEO of the Charles A. Dana Foundation. But he didn't see his primary mission as the giving-away of money; rather, he became an active advocate of a big idea.

Mahoney's idea was to awaken Americans to the potential of brain science and to focus public attention on its support. As recounted in this book, his message to the scientists assembled in the lab at Cold Spring Harbor was troubling and challenging: they were losing valuable years, and falling behind in funding, because they were failing to reach outside their scientific world. To enlist public support in a time of declining budgets and competing interests, he told them they would have to communicate—in understandable terms—the excitement in their field. "Nobody buys research," he told them, "but everybody buys hope." In marketing terms, they had to offer people not just intermittent reports of research, but hope—specific hope about how and when their work on the brain would cure diseases and improve people's lives. "These hopeful people want to know, in concrete terms, how you are going to help them; only then will they help you." This was met at first with narrowed eyes. Scientists resist hyperbole; they rightly look askance at promoters who prematurely announce "breakthroughs."

Then some of the scientists began to examine their own realistic expectations—advances they were confident could be accomplished in the foreseeable, short-term future. They identified the diseases of the brain, afflicting millions, that most people did not realize could be treated or conquered soon. At the marketing man's urging, they listed ten specific goals—realistic projections of breakthroughs to come, with concentrated effort—and set their signatures on a declaration that laid their own hopes and judgments on the line.

That started the Dana Alliance for Brain Initiatives, now an association of nearly 250 of the field's leaders, including an active sister organization just begun in Europe. Scientists once leery of public appearances are now more comfortable with seminars and interviews, and are also more familiar with one another's work. Journalists are finding these researchers and doctors far more accessible and ready to explain their work understandably.

Philanthropies and political bodies are being exposed to the potential for saving lives and saving billions in years ahead. And the general public is beginning to get the idea that the array of brain diseases—from Alzheimer's to stroke to brain cancer to depression to hundreds of others—need not be part of every person's future as we grow older.

"Hope moves people to invest in wider and more intensified research," says David now, still selling hard, "which in turn can justify their hope. We're seeing the results already." Several of the goals set at Cold Spring Harbor have been achieved; none of the scientists needed further urging from a marketing man to set fresh goals. That's why Jim Watson said recently that "David Mahoney is the Mary Lasker of this generation."

What made Mrs. Lasker the preeminent philanthropist of her day in the field of medical science and public health? It was not the amount of money she gave or raised. What made her count was the influence she brought to bear, by virtue of good judgment; a feel for the future of medicine; and the ability to transmit her enthusiasm to more cautious givers. Her husband, Albert Lasker, made his fortune as head of the Lord and Thomas advertising agency before turning to public service and philanthropy; a half century later, David Mahoney is using that same strategic marketing background to energize private and public support of brain science. (I can attest to that from personal experience: he roped me into serving as a Dana Foundation director years ago, and now I'm touting neuroscience research every chance I get, including this one.)

With every solution comes a problem. Suppose our hopes are realized. Suppose the physicians of the body, as we expect, lengthen our lives by curing the diseases that kill so many in our middle years. Suppose, too, that the neuroscientists come up with ways to extend memory and regenerate brain cells, not only keeping us alert but showing us how to use our minds to exert a positive influence on the health of our bodies. What then? What do we do in that extra generation of active life? Go fishing? Go to pot? Go broke? Go batty with boredom? Or go into a losing battle with a younger generation ready and eager to take power?

We need to have a strategy. All the amazing imaging techniques that let us begin to see the way we think must be fitted into a bigger picture. As David Mahoney and Dr. Richard Restak worked in many of these fields, they began to see the need for a comprehensive approach that each individual can take to gain the benefits that come from grasping the potential of becoming a centenarian. They took the separate strands that lead to the newly achievable longevity—good mental health habits, stress management, physical exercise and nutrition, dual-career development, and long-range financial planning—and wove them into "the Longevity Strategy."

That does not mean this book is more-holistic-than-thou. The authors take their subject seriously, but I'm glad they make a point about the mental and physical benefits of good humor (Mahoney was once the top Good Humor Man) and they know the need to lighten up now and then. "I don't want to achieve immortality through my work," said the philosopher Woody Allen. "I want to achieve immortality by not dying."

That's not part of the strategy, but this is: organize your life and your work around the possibility that you could live to 100. Granted, it's now a long shot, but the odds are coming down every day. The authors say: Your sensible preparations for a fourth quarter, and your positive attitude toward the real possibility of longer life, will enliven and enrich your every day. You don't have to be a brain scientist to figure out why that makes sense. Use your head.

William Safire

INTRODUCTION

WHEN YOU FINISH READING *The Longevity Strategy* you will have everything you will need to know to increase your chances of becoming a vigorous centenarian—living to be 100 years old and liking it.

Over the next 221 pages we will tell you how to employ scientifically sound tactics for achieving mental vigor, security, and health—to succeed in living long and happily. Thanks to the enormous recent gains in neuroscience, medicine, psychology, economics, nutrition, and health, such a goal is now possible. Scientists are becoming convinced that longevity depends on a dynamic interplay involving three factors: the health of our brain, our attitudes and thinking patterns, and our general health—in other words, the brain-body connection.

Especially important are research insights from all over the world that pinpoint the importance of the brain in keeping us healthy, recovering from illness, and improving both longevity and its quality. Indeed, new knowledge about the brain is the cornerstone of the longevity strategy.

We're not talking here about mind over matter. Rather, we suggest that by learning about your brain and applying that knowledge in your everyday life, you will increase your power to have and enjoy longevity.

Over many years, both of us have thought a lot about longevity. During those years we have enjoyed the privilege of a special access and exposure to world-class scientists and their research. By incorporating their knowledge with our own thoughts and insights, we have come up with a longevity strategy based on the brain and body's interaction.

The strategy comprises a life plan based on three objectives leading to a happy, healthy longevity:

- an optimally functioning brain in a sound body
- favorable social support systems
- financial security

The idea is to help you act as a potential centenarian—whatever your age at this moment—because the dedicated centenarian has a lot to do. This involves not only health matters but also decisions about how to proceed in key areas of life, ranging from the familial to the financial.

We can't stress enough: Science and medicine are far ahead of the usual views of aging. As you read this book, you'll realize that you have the power to redefine aging as joyfully spending—not being ravaged by—the gift of more time to do all that's important to you.

Here, set out in a series of short chapters, are the rules to follow to have the best chance of achieving what all of us place at the pinnacle of our wish list: how to live long and healthily and securely.

Before giving you those rules, just a few words about how this book came about and why, from time to time, we will refer to one of ourselves by name, as we do below, as if speaking about someone else.

On May 16, 1996, David Mahoney delivered the commencement address at Rutgers University. The speech, which he called "The Centenarian Strategy," was one of the first public occasions to focus on what, within a year, would start turning into a major topic of public discussion: the idea that science and medicine were making the 100-year life span possible, especially for those who are in their twenties and thirties today. David told the graduates that they should anticipate being hale and hearty to age 100 and beyond. Their minds will remain sound and sharp largely thanks to brain research and an increased awareness of brain health. David promised the graduates that if they follow a conscious centenarian strategy they will enjoy a lifetime of meaning, contribution, and satisfaction: "a lifetime of alertness that lasts a whole century."

After reading the speech, Richard Restak was intrigued with David's centenarian strategy. Later, in late 1996, David and Richard met for the first time, and after only a few moments they discovered they shared the conviction that medical research, especially *brain* research, is transforming "exceptional" longevity into the future norm.

Already there are indications that a prolonged longevity is upon us. Approximately one fifth of all of the people in the recorded history of the world who have ever lived to sixty-five years of age or older are alive right now. In short, "exceptional" longevity is no longer exceptional. The question is becoming, "What should I do to take advantage of this opportunity to live longer and healthier than any generation in history?"

At the time of the Mahoney-Restak meeting, David Mahoney was completing his nineteenth year as chairman and CEO of the Charles A. Dana Foundation, the most influential independent advocate of brain research in the world.

David is known to brain researchers internationally for the bold and provocative challenge he issued in 1992 at an international conference held at Cold Spring Harbor on Long Island, NY. In his address to James Watson, the famed geneticist and the meeting's organizer, and a veritable "college of cardinals" of the neuroscience community, David galvanized his distinguished audience.

Mahoney dared the eminent neuroscientists in the audience to "put their hands in the fire" and come up with objectives that could reasonably be achieved in brain research before the arrival of the third millennium.

At first the scientists didn't take to David's suggestion. They were resistant to the notion that they should actively seek public support. Shouldn't the public leave science to the scientists? David responded by telling them that if they were too proud to make a case for public support, they didn't deserve that support. The turning point in the meeting came when James Watson said, in so many words, that Mahoney was on to something here.

David then told them to speak clearly, say what they were doing, not to muffle their voices, and get it done *now*. He told his audience to come up with the scientific initiatives that they thought would make enormous progress over the next decade so he could bring them to the public.

In a heartfelt expression of confidence, the neuroscientists at Cold Spring Harbor took up the Mahoney challenge. They affixed their names to a declaration that, within the neuroscience community, would soon be compared, in terms of its importance to brain research, to a declaration of interdependence. These eminent brain scientists wrote:

We the undersigned, in order to commemorate the objectives of the Decade of the Brain; celebrate the achievements and bright future of neuroscience research; better understand, treat, and ultimately prevent brain disease; galvanize support for and stimulate public awareness of brain research; and enrich human life, do ordain and establish the Dana Alliance for Brain Initiatives.

"The bottom line is this: nothing that is going on in the world is as important as research into the diseases of—and into the positive potential of—the human brain," says David Mahoney. "We must always keep in mind what our efforts are about. They're about conquering disease and creating hope for patients and their families. They're about discovering how to end suffering and help us take care of each other."

Richard Restak's career up to the time of his meeting with

David Mahoney was also deeply involved with the brain. A neurologist and neuropsychiatrist, Richard became convinced early in his career that the general public would be fascinated with the brain if they only knew more about it.

In his writing Richard has sought to inform a wide range of readers about the brain. His contributions have ranged from best-selling books to publications on how brain damage affects everyday behavior to vignettes on how we can deepen our understanding of modern life by learning as much as we can about the brain. In his book *The Brain Has a Mind of Its Own*, Richard wrote of the brain processes underlying experiences as varied as philosophical speculation and why, once you learn, you never forget how to ride a bicycle.

On the basis of their shared interest in the human brain and their shared conviction that the advent of centenarian longevity will be the gift of the twentieth century to the twenty-first, David and Richard decided to work together on a unique project. Over many conversations they elaborated, extended, and refined David's "Centenarian Strategy" speech to a clear set of rules to help people live to 100 years of age or older. Based on their different backgrounds and experiences, they aimed at reconciling for the general reader their different insights drawn from the world of neuroscience and the world of business. The fruit of their collaboration is this book.

Their very different personal backgrounds are why David and Richard decided that, when they draw upon those backgrounds, they should tell you whose experience is being used. Obviously, "I" wouldn't be very helpful with two authors, and "we" wouldn't do when mentioning an experience that just one of them had. Thus they settled on the third-person device of "David" and "Richard"—which they hope helps keep things clear.

With this as general background, let's get down to the rules that form the foundation for the Longevity Strategy.

PART ONE

Get the Longevity Attitude

S*tart looking forward to living to 100 years of age or older. The twenty-first century will be the age of the centenarian.*

WHEN WILLARD SCOTT of NBC-TV started announcing 100th birthdays in 1980, only a handful of people applied for the honor of having their birthday celebrated on national television. Today he gets hundreds of letters a month. These letters are from members of the country's most exclusive club: individuals with authenticated life spans of more than 100 years. And that club is going to be taking in many more new members in coming decades.

Those who are eighty-five or older now constitute the fastest-growing population in the United States. There are now more than 60,000 members of the 100-plus club. By the year 2020 analysts predict that more than 200,000 Americans will be 100 years old or older.

We asked researchers at Bonn University in Germany who are studying longevity to list for us the important factors in reaching a healthy 100 years of age. Lists aren't the way to think about longevity, they informed us. Instead, they suggested thinking about interactive patterns involving personality, intelligence, and behavior. Included as components of those are activity, mood, adjustment, and social contact.

Sure, genetics plays a part: None of us exists without some genetic predisposition to one thing or another. But longevity does not seem to be heavily influenced by our genes. In addition, what we put down to genetics is often the result of complex social interactions.

In one study of longevity, two populations with "genetic" differences in longevity turned out to differ from each other in ways we all readily recognize: diet, levels of physical activity, and national and ethnic antistress rituals. But even more significantly, the researchers found regional longevity affected by "national and ethnic traditions—that is, respectful attitude toward the elderly, involvement in bringing up children and in the solution of familial and even regional problems."

Likewise, researchers at the University of Georgia Centenarian Study in Athens, Georgia, find that life satisfaction and health make up two interrelated components of adaptation. These include cognitive skills, life events and coping, activities, awareness/reminiscence, time use, and health-seeking behavior. A two-way communication exists between these adaptation characteristics and physical and mental health, which, in turn, influences longevity. But to increase longevity, it's necessary to understand the process of aging.

For years scientists have debated about the causes of aging. Two major theories compete for favor.

The first theory, "programmed senescence," is based on the belief that aging results from a genetic program. According to this theory, a person's life span depends on processes that begin at conception and extend over a given number of years. Implicit in this theory is the idea that longevity can be prolonged if scientists can discover the nature and functioning of the "biological clock"—the senescence program—that sets the outer limits on how long we can live.

The second theory holds that aging is a consequence of the random accumulation of errors brought about by chemical processes—principally the generation of unstable molecules known as free radicals. To achieve stability, free radicals steal electrons from DNA molecules. According to this theory, aging results from the ensuing damage to DNA throughout the body.

Both theories of aging are at least partly true. Programmed senescence can be seen in the different life expectancies observed from one species to another irrespective of health or lifestyle: no dog or cat has ever lived for 100 years. But even within the same species, the life span can differ greatly: some dogs live a lot longer than others. This variation in life span is at least partially a reflection of differences in life experience, including the effects of free radicals and other chemicals on cell functioning.

In short, longevity in an individual can be analyzed statistically but not predicted precisely. That's because longevity in the individual involves an inherent randomness that defies prediction. The statistical and actuarial tables used by insurance companies are based on this randomness. According to these tables, certain habits, such as smoking and excessive drinking, can be shown to shorten the average life span in a population. But statistical tables do not allow predictions of mortality in a specific person, as they could if longevity were primarily genetically determined.

"People aren't likely to live long just because their parents did," according to Leonard Poon, who heads the University of Georgia's Centenarian Study. "It seems the genetic contribution is important for some centenarians who come from a long line of long-lived people. But we have as many [centenarians] who do not come from long-lived families."

After studying more than 150 centenarians who have volunteered for the study, Poon is in an excellent position to know that good genes can only do so much toward helping you reach 100.

Like most of the researchers we know who study aging, Poon has concluded that extreme longevity results from the interplay of many different factors, among them several surprises. One is that his findings do not support the widespread popular belief that consuming—or avoiding—certain foods promotes longevity.

Why do we think Poon did not discern a dietary component to longevity? Centenarians grew into maturity during periods when less was known about the benefits of a good diet and the negative health consequences of a bad one. The majority of people in that generation who ate the same diet never reached the age of 100. The take-home lesson is this: The body does the best it can with whatever we put into our mouths. But if we are wiser about the foods we eat, our body has an easier time of it and, as a secondary benefit, our chances for enhanced longevity are increased.

In support of this, centenarians in Poon's study, whatever their diet, typically eat a wide variety of vegetables and take in more vitamin A and carotenoids than in a control group of sixty- and eighty-year-olds. Moreover, many of the centenarians are now reversing some of their past unwise dietary choices. Poon and the nutritionist involved in the study, Mary Ann Johnson, found out that about 50 percent of centenarians in their group try now to avoid fats in their diets.

An additional surprise concerned the personality of the typical centenarian. Forget about the lamblike dispositions and beatific smiles of the stereotypical oldster you're likely to encounter on a television commercial. Compared with younger groups, the centenarians are determined overall to have their own way. "They tend to be independent: they tend to dominate—they want their own way," Poon says. "As a result of living 100 years or more, centenarians have a wide variety of experiences behind them and have outlived spouses, friends, even their own children. Experts on the art of survival, centenarians score high on optimism; they are rarely depressed."

While centenarians share many things in common, differences outweigh similarities. Poon found his subjects differ in social and economic levels, education, work experience, religious beliefs, and level of prosperity. This, of course, is worth celebrating: it means that nobody has an exclusive on the chance to live until 100.

A different study—the New England Centenarian Study—has also discovered something surprising. According to Thomas T. Perls, principal investigator of this study, "The centenarians I have met have, with few exceptions, reported that their nineties were essentially problem-free. As nonagenarians, many were employed, sexually active, and enjoyed the outdoors and the arts."

Perls has observed that, after age ninety-seven, a person's chance of dying tends to veer from the expected trend and actually becomes reduced. This supports his theory that the "oldest old" tend to be healthier than is traditionally believed. For reasons that no one understands, "Some people are particularly resistant to acquiring the disorders that disable and kill most people before age ninety. Because of this resistance, they not only outlive others, they do so relatively free of infirmities." The key question is, of course: how do they do that?

No single factor stands out. Rather, reaching 100 years of age depends on a combination of factors. These include: a genetic makeup that predisposes to long survival; a positive attitude toward life; good stress-coping skills; health-promoting behaviors that reduce the risk of getting sick; sufficient common sense to deal with everyday problems of living; and, finally, the good fortune to avoid infectious diseases and serious injuries.

Can we really learn anything from people who were born before the first airplane flew, before women had the vote, before income taxes, before vitamins were known about? Yes, we can learn deliberately what they knew intuitively: centenarians possess an intuitive knowledge of the difference between aging and becoming old. The difference? Becoming old means:

- losing interest in life
- accepting the notion that it's too late to change
- believing that life doesn't matter anymore
- failing to set goals and commitments
- losing a sense of surprise and giving in to boredom

None of us can stop aging, but we don't have to grow old.

CHAPTER 2

Discard negative stereotyped thinking about aging.

CARDINAL SPELLMAN ONCE SAID, "The three ages of man are youth, middle age, and 'You're looking wonderful.'" The remark was ironic then, but today it's true and getting truer.

On March 25, 1997, former president George Bush, at age seventy-three, gave a very public demonstration of the kinds of things older people can accomplish. A 12,500-foot sky dive over the Arizona desert is an impressive feat for anyone, no matter his or her age.

Three months after Bush's sky dive, Mary Fasano, age eighty-nine, graduated from Harvard University. She is the oldest person to earn a Harvard degree in its 361 years.

U.S. Senator John Glenn, the first American to orbit the Earth, revealed, after announcing his retirement from the Senate, that he was talking to NASA about going back into space. The space agency said Glenn wants to go again, not for nostalgia, but to further studies of bone loss in aging, using what they've learned about its occurrence in weightlessness. He is age seventy-six.

These three vigorous individuals, along with increasing

numbers of lesser-known septuagenarians and octogenarians, represent the future of aging in America.

Between 1960 and 1990 the overall U.S. population grew 39 percent. While those under twenty-five increased by 13 percent, the ranks of those eighty-five or older leaped 232 percent. The over-sixty-five group nearly doubled, increasing by 89 percent. Accompanying this explosion is a major change in the health of older people.

Soon feats such as those of George Bush, Mary Fasano, and Glenn will become commonplace because the seventy-plus segment of our nation's population has never been healthier.

Disability rates in Americans older than sixty-five dropped 15 percent between 1982 and 1994, according to scientists at the Duke University Center for Demographic Studies. Smarter, healthier living is responsible for this improvement, according to Kenneth G. Manton, the professor who oversees the Duke study—and that is without factoring in recent medical advances, a question Manton is now studying.

But physical health is only part of the picture. How satisfied are older people about the quality of their lives?

To find out, a researcher in Finland, Dr. Minna K. Eronen, followed, for ten years, 241 women between ages fifty and sixty. Rather than feeling worse with the passage of time, these women felt better. The women rating their physical fitness as good or fairly good increased from about one in four in 1982 to almost a third in 1992. When asked to compare their present life satisfaction with that of five years earlier, 37 percent reported greater satisfaction, 29 percent felt there had been no change, while only 34 percent felt their life situation had worsened. In another survey, carried out in 1976, older people turned out to be far happier than most of us believe. Only 7 percent of those Finns surveyed reported feeling lonely most of the time; only 8 percent felt that they had nothing to look forward to.

"These findings suggest that some positive changes may take place in women's quality of life as they age from their fifties into their sixties," according to Dr. Eronen. "These positive changes should be publicized so that women approaching retirement age do not need to worry unnecessarily about the quality of life in their latter years."

Those numbers don't surprise David's wife, Hillie: "As I grow older, I find it easier to keep an open mind about things and keep growing. Balance and proportion come easier. If things are good, you're more joyful because you're more centered. If things aren't so good, you realize that 'this, too, shall pass.'"

Too often, our ideas about aging are not only inaccurate but also often involve hurtful and destructive stereotypes that need to be recognized and eliminated. "We often unconsciously buy into stereotypes that define people by age," according to Carolyn Restak, Richard's wife, a mother of three daughters and a specialist in conducting clinical trials of new brain drugs. "Aging stereotypes negatively affect us all. If you age-stereotype, you miss out on a wealth of information and knowledge that you can learn only from mature people. We have to learn to be age-blind."

One of the most pervasive stereotypes involves physical appearance. Ask a random group of people if they consider good looks as a factor in their determinations about the mental spryness of an older person. Your respondents will tell you that they don't even take physical attractiveness into consideration. Yet psychological experiments show just the opposite: attractive younger people are often perceived as mentally sharper and more "with it" than older people who are not especially good-looking. We've all seen too many movies. In real life the heroes and heroines can't be identified by their looks.

Another example of stereotyped thinking about aging

emerged from a survey, Images of Aging in America, conducted by the American Association of Retired Persons in 1994. Twelve hundred older adult Americans were asked to rate their concerns about crime, insufficient money, loneliness, poor health, and other social factors, such as the sense of being needed and of keeping busy. They then were asked: "How serious a problem do you think these things are for most people over sixty-five these days?" The results showed a much higher estimate of such problems in *other* older people than in the respondents themselves. For instance, while not having enough money was a problem for only 12 percent of the respondents, they considered insufficient money likely to be a problem for 55 percent of other people over sixty-five.

Other stereotypes frequently creep into the thinking of older people about themselves. For instance, Becca Levy, Ph.D., of Harvard University has found that older people show dramatic memory improvement when the negative stereotypes of aging that dominate our culture are modified.

Levy discovered that if she could change these negative stereotypes into more positive ideas about aging, the memory performance of older people would improve along with their sense of control.

She did this by reminding older individuals of the wisdom traditionally associated with aging, their greater experience, and their enhanced ability to integrate a lifetime of accumulated knowledge. But if she said or implied things consistent with negative stereotyping (e.g., mentioning that older people are naturally more forgetful), memory performance fell off and, along with it, the older person's sense of control and general attitude toward aging. Thus memory performance can be influenced in a positive way simply on the basis of the attitudes older people are encouraged to hold about themselves.

That's why it's necessary to learn as much as you can about the aging process. Many of the anxieties we all hold about growing older diminish with knowledge and understanding. We commend to you what the essayist M. F. K. Fisher wrote when "well into" her seventies:

"Parts of the Aging Process are scary, of course, but the more we know about them, the less they need be. That is why I wish we were more deliberately taught, in early years, to prepare for this condition. It would leave a lot of us freed to enjoy the obvious rewards of being old, when the sound of a child's laugh, or the catch of sunlight on a flower petal is as poignant as ever was a girl's voice to an adolescent ear, or the tap of a golfball into its cup to a balding banker's. . . . We are unprepared for the years that may come as our last ones. . . . Plainly, I think that this clumsy modern pattern is a wrong one, an ignorant one, and I regret and wish that I could do more to change it."

One way of changing this pattern involves learning about the physical, mental, and emotional changes that occur with aging. One impediment to doing this, of course, is our fear that everything we will learn about aging will fit into the general category of bad news. But as we will develop further in this book, research contradicts this dire and overly pessimistic assumption.

CHAPTER 3

A ssume the odds are in your favor.
If we all discard our stereotyped ideas
about aging, the question about
longevity comes down to this: Is it
reasonable to plan to live to be 100?
What are the odds?

UNTIL RECENTLY MOST SCIENTISTS thought that genetics
made it unlikely that the human life span could be routinely
extended to 100. That's because most scientists, like most other
people, rarely encountered centenarians. What's more, there
was often good reason to doubt the accuracy of the birth records
of many of those claiming to have reached the century mark.

Today, with more careful record keeping, we know that
many healthy 100-year-olds exist. On February 21, 1997, Jeanne
Calment, who was officially the world's oldest person, celebrated
her 122nd birthday. She died later that year, the oldest person in
history whose age could be verified by official documents.

But documenting the existence of a Mme. Calment (and thereby raising the possibility that many more of us could become centenarians) is only part of the battle. To make such longevity a common event in the twenty-first century and beyond, all of us will have to adopt necessary lifestyle changes. We already know many of the things that are killing us, but eliminating them isn't turning out to be as simple as it first seemed.

For one thing, we have to overcome the tendency to put too much emphasis on our genetic inheritance. We have to stop blaming our genes for our health and longevity. While it's true that genetics plays a part in our susceptibility to certain diseases, which may thereby shorten our life, heredity accounts for only about one quarter of the variation in human life spans.

Scientists have investigated the role of genes in longevity by studying twins. One of these studies—of twins born in Denmark and tracked over many years by government records—reveals no evidence that genes set the life span. Instead, they make it more (or less) likely that a subject will come down with life-shortening diseases such as Alzheimer's disease, cancer, or heart disease. This distinction carries important practical consequences.

If the life span were simply set by a gene, then the only way of increasing longevity would be to somehow alter the action of that gene (or genes if more than one were involved). But since genes code much more for diseases rather than life span—and diseases can be cured, prevented, or at least delayed—longevity can be increased through medical advances. Indeed, that is what has happened over the past several decades.

Thanks to medical breakthroughs and healthier lifestyles, life expectancy has increased by three or four years each decade. Included here are dramatic reductions in infant mortality along with reductions of deaths and illnesses secondary to heart disease and stroke—the latter two made possible by better control of blood pressure and other risk factors. And we have lens implants, hip and knee replacements, and other prosthetic devices that only a few years ago were the stuff of medical science fiction. All of these have resulted in a declining disability rate and a twenty-eight-year gain in life expectancy since 1928.

Today we can expect to live to 75.5 years, up from 47 at the start of the twentieth century. At the moment, the 3.8 million people 85 or older are the fastest-growing segment of the population. Over the next two or three decades, decreases in chronic disability, coupled with breakthroughs in our ability to cure and prevent disabling illnesses, should push the average life span well into the eighties by 2030. In other words, soon we will be just as shocked to hear that someone died at 67 as we are now when we hear that a person died at 47.

An estimate for Western Europe published in the journal *Nature* in the early 1990s concluded that as medical advances further increase life expectancy, the proportion of people over sixty will double to 20 percent by 2050 and reach 27 percent by 2100. And in America? The U.S. Census Bureau expects our eighty-five-plus group to more than double, to 9 million, by 2030.

Bear in mind that, for a person to be eighty-five in 2030, he or she is now fifty-two, well into middle age. In other words, we think this makes all the projections conservative, because the octogenarian of 2030 grew to adulthood without the benefit of many of the health insights we now take for granted: the perils of smoking, too much fat in the diet, and physical inactivity weren't nearly as well publicized from 1950 through 1980 as they are today.

What's more, people who will be eighty-five or older two decades later, in 2050, are now in their midthirties. Because they learned more as they grew up about how to promote health and prevent disease, their chances of reaching eighty-five or older are even greater.

But why cap the life span at eighty-five? Many credible scientists believe today's newborns will live on average to 100. Part of their optimism is based on the advances that can be expected in our ability to control and cure many of the killing diseases that prevent us from reaching the centenarian age. If present health measures are combined with expected health advances over the next decade, such as new medications and additional lifestyle changes, living to 100 might become far more commonplace.

Three demographers (students of human populations) from Duke University and Yale University have developed a model that assesses the effect of present and future health trends on longevity. They applied their model to more than 5,000 participants in a health study that ran from 1950 to 1984. The demographers claim, based on their model, that if the participants in the health study had been keeping blood pressure and cholesterol and other risk factors at normal levels for a typical 30-year-old, the men would have lived to an average of 99.9 years.

Nor are such predictions unrealistic. Death from heart disease fell 71 percent between 1958 and 1992, and stroke and other forms of vascular disease also decreased to a lesser extent. But the most dramatic health change in the past twenty years has involved diet. As recently as a decade ago, almost all of us were eating and drinking too much. Many of us smoked; few of us did much exercise. While a decade is too short a time to measure an effect on longevity, you can be sure that these health improvements are going to have an effect, and a powerful one—not that the effects can be guaranteed to be simple or straightforward.

Take smoking, for instance. We don't know many reasonably informed people over forty who still smoke cigarettes. There is simply too much information that cannot be ignored on how cigarettes can kill you. But despite the ready availability of damning information about smoking, the habit is making a rebound among twenty- and thirty-year-olds, perhaps because smoking cigarettes is associated in their minds with rebellion and individual expression.

Whatever the cause, a paradox exists: while diet and exercise guidelines are being followed, the most important health insight of all is being largely ignored. This paradox has the potential to exert a major negative impact on the younger generation's chances of living to be centenarians. Rather than despairing, however, we're confident that with a different informational approach emphasizing how "uncool" smoking really is, people of all ages will give up the habit.

If you or somebody you know and love still smokes, you should ponder the findings of Drs. Christopher J. L. Murray of the Harvard School of Public Health and Alan D. Lopez of the World Health Organization. These doctors calculated trends in death and disability through the years 1990 to 2020. They concluded that tobacco-related deaths would offset the gains science is making against noncommunicable diseases. In fact, they project that tobacco use could be the "largest single health problem in 2020."

Translation: If you smoke and plan to continue to do so, you might as well stop reading right here and cancel your goal of becoming a centenarian. This is not a book about miracles.

CHAPTER 4

Develop the correct mental attitudes now to improve your chances of being a centenarian.

SOME INTRIGUING RESEARCH shows that conscientiousness (social dependability) in childhood predicts longevity. This finding is incredible when you think about it: childhood personality is related to survival decades into the future! What could account for such an association? Nobody has it figured out yet, but there is a lot of expert speculation.

Perhaps "conscientious" people are more careful about avoiding overeating, alcohol, and cigarettes. Maybe they take fewer risks and as a result get into fewer fatal accidents.

While these explanations sound reasonable, they haven't held up to careful analysis correlating the causes for people's death with known risk factors for early death such as tobacco and alcohol abuse.

When researchers from the Department of Psychology at the University of California in Riverside looked at the question, they decided that conscientiousness must work in additional, less obvious, but wide-ranging ways to affect health and longevity.

Not that any of this should come as a surprise, in our opinion. Becoming a centenarian, or at least doing everything you can to achieve it, is a lifetime enterprise. A conscientious person sets goals for himself or herself and carries through with those goals. Such a person recognizes obligations not just to himself or herself but to others as well.

To learn more about the secrets of living well, Richard spoke to Stanley Jacobson, a longtime friend and colleague. Jacobson, a seventy-five-year-old clinical psychologist, has for several years led a group—whom he calls "vital agers"—of about a dozen men and women ranging in age from their midsixties to nearly ninety. All of the members of Jacobson's group are solidly committed to living full lives. Richard asked Jacobson about his group's secrets to growing old.

Jacobson said that there aren't any secrets, just several traits he's observed that are possessed by those who are aging gracefully.

- *Basic optimism.* They enjoy fellowship, relish new experience, live one day at a time toward a future that may be limited in duration but not in richness.

- *Willingness to adapt.* Whatever the challenges, vital agers learn to circumvent the disabilities where they can and to accept the limits they cannot overcome.

- *Sense of personal power and readiness to take responsibility.* They actively search for solutions to the problems we face in health, housing and financing or retirement.

- *Resilience.* This is the ability to bounce back from misfortune.

- *Involvement in meaningful projects and relationships.* All vital agers are engaged in life. They have work to do and they pursue it with energy and purpose.

- *Healthy self-esteem.* This is perhaps the most important of all the keys to vital aging. Americans with this trait pursue their projects and relationships with a confidence in the validity of their endeavors. Whether the world wants to know it or not, vital agers know that they can govern their own lives.

Those traits will not only increase your chances of becoming a centenarian but also will provide a framework for everyday living.

Psychiatrists frequently speak about rescue fantasies, and we all have them. If you smoke, or drink too much, or act irresponsibly, chances are you retain in your imagination a scenario where you are rescued at the last moment from the consequences of your behavior. Such fantasies aren't abnormal. They are a residue from early childhood when somebody, usually Mom or Dad, did come to our rescue. Maybe they told us what to say to an overly demanding playmate or straightened something out with a teacher. But in regard to your present physical and mental well-being, nobody can come to your rescue except yourself.

Among the behaviorally influenced factors important in longevity and health are: smoking, alcohol and drug consumption, diet and activity, exposure to toxins and microorganisms, involvement with firearms, personal safety precautions, safe sexual behavior, and motor vehicle accidents. We have some control over all of these. But only we can exercise this control; nobody can do it for us.

If there's one "umbrella" mental attitude for the aspiring centenarian, it is to remember that biology isn't destiny. As Jeanette Ickovics, assistant professor of medicine and psychology at Yale University, says, "Genes contribute no more than 25 percent to our health, while the environment and our behavior provide the additional 75 percent. Indeed, one half of all deaths can be attributed to behaviors rather than something just 'happening' to us. It's what you do and what you think that matter the most."

The goal is to achieve what Jeanette Ickovics calls *allostasis:* stability through change. Allostasis concentrates on the dynamism that characterizes the human body and mind. This dynamism extends even to the level of our genes. One of the pivotal insights of the past decade is that genes are not immutable, not one and forever particles of heredity that are passed down from parents to children, like family jewels. The action of genes changes according to the environment and according to behavior. We know this from the study of how the new antidepressants work.

Neuropsychiatrists have known for years that depression doesn't begin to lift fully until several weeks after starting an antidepressant. What is happening during that time? The anti-depressant is altering the genes' activity so that different enzymes and neurotransmitters spring into action. The brain is literally altered by the medication in ways that depend on gene modification.

This new and exciting idea, that the activity of genes can be modified, provides hope where there was, until only recently, a good deal of despair. After all, if "it's all in the genes" and "genes can't be altered," what sense would there be to try to make changes in our lives? But the truth is just the opposite: only we can make changes that have the potential to help make us centenarians. The rule is simplicity itself: eliminate health-damaging behavior while enhancing health-promoting behaviors.

Remember what Cary Grant said: "If I had known I was going to live this long, I would have taken better care of myself."

PART TWO

The Long-Living Brain

CHAPTER 5

Start learning now as much as you can about your brain. While we will live longer than any generation in history, the major advances in longevity in our lifetime are going to come from brain research.

NOBEL PRIZE WINNER James Watson once said, "Someday we are going to be proud of our brains, instead of just a little bit afraid of them." Thanks to brain research we are already replacing fear and ignorance with pride and knowledge.

The Longevity Strategy means that you will do a lot more with that pride and knowledge than just luxuriate in them. You're going to:

- want to tweak those high-performing parts of your brain so you're always leading with your strengths
- relax—a lot—about normal slips and trips of the brain as you get older

- become good at calibrating the loads you give your brain to handle

- be more tolerant of quirks in your friends and loved ones

- start giving your brain support in its job of "controller" for your body

- discover how to tell your doctor about symptoms that just might be information from your brain about a problem *it* has

- discover that you understand the brain-related information your doctor tells you he's getting from your symptoms

- appreciate why each of us is different, and yet we all have the same opportunity for a long and fulfilling life

You will probably think of many more benefits by the time you've finished this book, but if you need any more convincing about the importance of the brain, let us suggest you ponder the following facts:

- Fifty million Americans—one person in five—suffer from diseases of the brain.

- Not all of us will develop cancer. Not all of us will get AIDS. Fortunately, not all of us will have a heart attack. But every one of us, at some time in our lives, will experience a brain or nervous system problem.

- Almost every family in America is touched by a brain-related disease, including Alzheimer's, Parkinson's, schizophrenia, or depression.

- The cost to society of these disorders of the brain and the nervous system is estimated to be well over $600 billion a year.

- Research in brain science is today making rapid strides and offers real promise for cures and prevention for the future.

A big cause of the speedup in findings about the brain is the invention of technology able to look into the living human brain at work—brain imaging, as it is called. Where the brain used to be a frustrating "black box" that scientists could inspect only after death, the new technologies let researchers see, rather than just deduce, brain processes as they occur. It is hard to overstate the contribution of imaging to longevity: it has added remarkable impetus to the development of effective diagnoses and treatments for many difficult brain disorders that shorten and damage the quality of life.

One of the most sensitive and revealing technologies, "positron emission tomography" or PET scanning, is now a diagnostic tool that you may experience sometime in your life. Under the prodding of legislation by Senator Ted Stevens of Alaska, the government has just approved Medicare and Medicaid reimbursement for PET scans, meaning that most private insurers are likely to follow suit.

PET tracks the blood sugar, glucose, by detecting a radioactive "tag" injected into the bloodstream. The brain consumes glucose in its operations, and PET registers areas of activity as bright spots on the brain image it creates. Aimed elsewhere in the body, PET detects cancers years before symptoms appear. The disorders for which scans will be covered are lung cancer, Alzheimer's disease, colorectal cancer, lymphomas, heart disease, and breast cancer. The Food and Drug Administration is also considering requiring pharmaceutical manufacturers to use PET to evaluate the safety of new drugs that may affect the brain.

One of the coinventors of PET, Dr. Mike Phelps of UCLA, predicts that PET scans will someday be routine in health checkups—with PET looking for changes in brain metabolism.

Metabolic change is the brain's first response, to compensate for a disease that has begun; you start to notice symptoms only after the disease overpowers this effort to fight back—often too late for treatment that might have helped earlier.

Phelps also feels that—apart from diagnosing disorders—PET scanning will give momentum to brain fitness for everyone interested in their own health. "I think PET will actually be a 'biofeedback' tool for the brain," he says. "We use all kinds of feedback to monitor our health; PET will reinforce us in doing the things we should do to improve our brain's functioning"— a kind of seeing-is-believing effect making us attentive to it. Phelps says this awareness is especially important because studies show that between ages twenty and eighty, the brain's metabolic rate does not decrease. "We sense a decline because some losses do take place, but the metabolic rate means the brain is ready to go. We need to exercise it, just like the body, to keep it fit as we age."

But the important research for the centenarian relates to what we have learned in the past few years about the brain as it ages. Forget about everything you've heard about brain cell loss. Actually, the brain doesn't lose cells in the thinking areas of the cerebral cortex. Nor is the brain of the older person an inferior version of his or her younger counterpart. Rather, the mature brain is organized differently, shows different strengths, and can remodel itself rather than "deteriorate" with age.

Research and new discoveries about the brain are particularly important because the human brain is our fundamental and essential human resource. All that we are and can ever be; everything that we think, including our inmost thoughts and dreams; every action we ever take or even consider taking—all of these are dependent on the brain. What's more, by knowing more about the brain, we can attain a kind of self-knowledge that can be applied in everyday situations. And by this we mean more than just from time to time; as you gain understanding of the crosstalk between brain and body, you will become better able to take advantage of your brain's partnership in your longevity.

For example, we all know vaguely that stress isn't good for our health. But now that simple insight has taken on new meaning. Within the past few years neuroscientists have discovered that hormones secreted in response to stress can damage the brain, leading to loss of volume in an area called the hippocampus, which plays an important role in learning and remembering. This discovery lifts the need for stress reduction above merely feeling better, and even above protecting our general health, all the way up to how we keep our memory and mental ability strong as we age. That's why we will give a whole chapter to stress and its management in this book.

You don't have to take a neurology residency to have a working knowledge of the brain. Despite its complexity, you can understand a lot if you know a few key facts and a handful of operating principles:

Imagine yourself sitting before a small stainless steel table on which sits a human brain (see Illustrations A, B, and C). What you see is a gray mass about the size of a grapefruit and divided into two hemispheres separated by a midline cleft that extends from the front of the brain to the back. If you put a gloved finger into the cleft and push down ever so gently you encounter a thick ligament, the corpus callosum, which connects the two hemispheres. The outer gray matter—the cortex—is less than five thousandths of an inch thick yet contains the millions of nerve cells that form the basis for our all-complex mental processes.

Just beneath the thin outer cortex of the hemispheres lies the brain's white matter. This is made up of closely connected fibers that join separate areas of the cortex, conduct impulses originating from the outside world to the brain, and redirect impulses in the opposite direction from the brain to the periphery. The white matter is a great coordinator of information within the brain. Longevity-associated disturbances in the white matter include strokes and damage done by the clogging of small blood vessels.

If you continue your exploration even deeper you will encounter additional islands of gray matter, the basal ganglia (see Illustration D). These subcortical nuclei assist in the appropriate planning, initiation, coordination, guidance, and termination of voluntary movements. Disturbances here result in age-associated diseases such as Parkinson's, which are marked by difficulties in the initiation or control of movement.

Another important deep structure, at the back of the brain, is the cerebellum. This is specialized for fine muscle and motor control. The performances of a concert pianist or a gymnast are dependent on the cerebellum working at its best. As we age, this area becomes less efficient, one of the reasons why you don't see many aging ballerinas. Cerebellar cell loss also helps explain why balance gets harder and why falls are more frequent with aging.

Digging still deeper, you approach the brain stem, composed of the midbrain, the pons, the medulla oblongata and, finally, the spinal cord, which can be thought of as an extension of the brain. The brain stem and spinal cord serve as conduits for the flow of nerve impulses to and from the brain. Chemical changes may occur along the brain stem, resulting mostly in age-associated depressions and disturbances of movement.

For years scientists believed that the brain, particularly the cerebral cortex, deteriorated with age. Contemporary research does not support such a gloomy outlook.

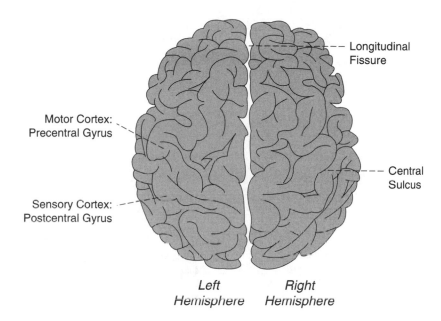

Illustration A.   *Hemispheres of the brain, seen from the top.* Adapted by Leigh Coriale Design and Illustration from *Brain, Mind and Behavior*, 2/E by F. Bloom and A. Lazerson © 1985, 1988 by Educational Broadcasting Corp. Used with permission.

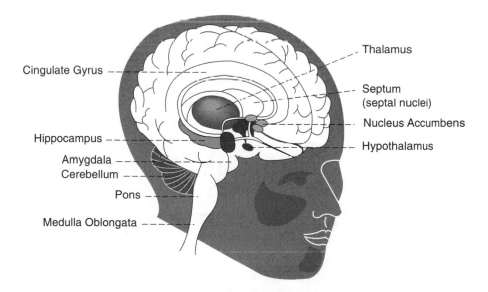

Illustration B.   *Major brain areas controlling thought, movement, and emotion—interior view.* Illustration by Leigh Coriale Design and Illustration.

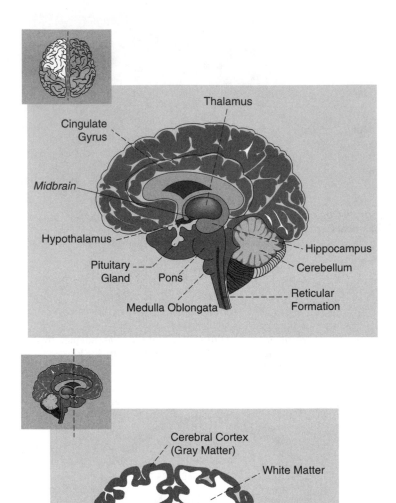

Illustrations C and D. Side and frontal views show other features important to longevity, including the hippocampus (a key memory area), the cerebellum (fine control of muscles and movement), and the basal ganglia (networks important in movement). Illustrations adapted by Leigh Coriale Design and Illustration from original illustrations by Patricia J. Wynne. Used with permission.

For one thing, neuroscientists agree that it's often difficult to separate normal aging from age-associated experiences. In comparison to a twenty-year-old, an eighty-year-old has had more exposure to alcohol, tobacco (passive smoke in nonsmokers), and other environmental pollutants. The eighty-year-old is also more likely to have experienced during those additional sixty years some form of head injury. How does one decide which differences in the eighty-year-old brain should be attributed to the passage of the years and which ones to those other harmful exposures?

In addition, it is incorrect to assume that a loss of neurons is necessarily a bad thing. Earlier in life the number of nerve cells in parts of the brain drops by as much as 30 percent. This is a normal process often equated to the art of sculpture.

"In a figurative sense, we might liken the loss of neuronal number to the chips that fall off from a slab of marble so that the underlying sculpture can emerge," according to M. Marsel Mesulam of the Cognitive Neurology and Alzheimer's Disease Center at Northwestern University Medical School in Chicago. Obviously there are limits to such an analogy. "In extreme aging or in diseased aging (for example, Alzheimer's disease), the falling chips begin to come from the sculpture itself," observes Mesulam. But in the normally aging brain, there is no correlation between mental powers and nerve cell numbers. That's why nerve cell counts alone can never provide a "gold standard" for assessing the normality of an older person's brain.

We cannot think of brain aging simply in terms of the number of brain cells still living. Loss of brain cells from the cerebrum, particularly from the all-important cortex, the outer five thousandths of an inch, varies widely from one person to another. Many neuroscientists are now convinced that the brain is capable of superior performance even into the tenth decade and beyond.

"In recent years as scientists have learned more about the processes of aging and the neurobiology and diseases of the aging brain, it has become apparent that the aging process does not, by itself, lead to dementia or degenerative diseases," says Zaven S. Khachaturian, director of the Alzheimer's Association's Ronald and Nancy Reagan Research Institute. "In the absence of disease, the human brain can and does continue to function unimpaired—often well into the tenth decade of life."

The implications of this new concept about the brain are amazing. If the brain remains healthy and doesn't fall prey to disease, then it should continue to function normally for as long as we live. Nerve cells should remain alive and maintain their connections. Even more important, nerve cells should be capable of forming new connections and forming networks throughout life.

To David, who as we write this is seventy-four, this is why we have to think of "living" when we think about "aging": "Our interests and our activities create new nerve pathways, revitalizing the brain and enhancing its functioning. In the past twelve years my neuronal connections have undergone profound changes as a result of my involvement with some of the most creative people in the world. This has not only been intellectually stimulating but also a great source of pleasure at the same time. Our brains thrive on stimulation. We're never happier than when we're extending our brain's capacities and learning something new."

Successful aging benefits not only the individual but our whole society as well. Thanks to having lived longer lives, older people have had the chance to see and learn more. Thus they are in a position to synthesize and update knowledge in many different areas. Succeeding generations benefit from the synthesizing and integrating capacities of the mature brain.

With maturity, our brains process information differently.

Think of it as a deepening and enriching process that culminates in what is traditionally described as wisdom. While wisdom can be found at any age, it usually requires a certain life experience, an experience that cannot be hurried. With advancing years, each of us has the opportunity of becoming older and wiser.

"Many societies have benefited from modes of governance where an attribute called wisdom, and usually distinguished from cleverness and intelligence, has been identified in old individuals," according to Dr. Mesulam.

At the moment, scientists lack an objective measure of wisdom. Psychological testing is no help here. A twenty-year-old may attain impressive scores on tests of memory, intelligence, and general mental performance, yet he or she may make a poor judge, negotiator, surgeon, or airline pilot. Don't we all daily encounter examples of this discrepancy between intelligence and wisdom?

But even if we can't always define wisdom, we can recognize it when we see it. This is particularly true when it comes to practical wisdom. David suggests we all strive for *seichel*, a Yiddish term for know-how, practical, everyday knowledge. His favorite example is Napoleon's mother.

David: "She could not understand why her son should take on the British and Wellington when things were going so well. But knowing he was going to do it anyway, she liquidated all of her French holdings and currency and converted them to British pounds. She did this based on the premise that if Napoleon won, she would have no problem in the victorious nation, but if he lost, as he did, she would not be wiped out. She had *seichel*."

Whether canny *seichel* or more profound wisdom, this quality is unique to each of us, because it is all that we've learned and experienced and has no exact location in the brain. But neuroscientists are getting a good idea of some of the processes that help in getting us there—and it's those processes that having and using a longevity strategy gives us the power to protect.

The Sociable Brain

We call brain science "neuroscience" because the fundamental unit of the human brain is the neuron. However many there are in the brain (a point of some disagreement among neuroscientists), the possible combinations of linkages of one neuron to another are nearly limitless.

The nerve cell or neuron is like a formula for corporate success: a design based on networking. A solitary neuron is as bereft of purpose and opportunity as a person stranded on a desert island. Our identity as social creatures is hardwired into the very structure of our brain. As we will see, this pattern of interconnectedness and sociability exists at every level of brain function.

Michael Gazzaniga is a neuroscientist famous for his work on the actions of the cerebral hemispheres. He says: "Our mental lives amount to a reconstruction of the independent activities of the many brain systems we all possess. A confederation of mental systems resides within us. Metaphorically, we humans are more of a sociological entity than a single unified psychological entity. We have a social brain."

At the basis of this sociability is the communication between and among neurons. This takes place by electrical and chemical means. Each neuron has a cell body, which like other cells in the body contains a nucleus and various supporting structures responsible for the synthesis of chemicals used in signaling. The neurons communicate with each other via a single axon and multiple dendrites.

The axon is a unique extension from the cell body that may travel only a few millimeters or, alternately, may extend a meter or more away. The axon conveys information by means of an electrical current called the "action potential," which propagates, rumorlike, from its point of origin at the cell body to its audience at the tip end of the axon. Once the message reaches the axon tip, it is converted from an electrical to a chemical message.

Neurotransmitters (chemical messengers) move across across a tiny gap (the synapse) separating neurons and latch on to special receptors like a lock and its key. This interaction of the neurotransmitter and its receptor results in widespread information throughout the brain. Psychopharmacologists have learned over the past three decades to treat mental and neurological illnesses (henceforth we'll call them neuropsychiatric disorders) by manipulating the levels of neurotransmitters in the synapse and their interactions with their receptors.

Researchers are now looking hard for ways to increase the healthy life span of the brain by the same chemical means. Some

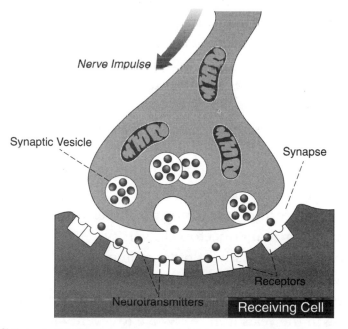

Socializing: A chemical message crosses the tiny gap (synapse) between neurons.
Altered from Kibiuk/Society for Neuroscience by Leigh Coriale Design and Illustration. Used with permission.

studies already show that chemically counteracting neuron loss from diseases that strike the aging brain is a plausible scenario.

For example, orally active compounds called *neuroimmunophilins* are proving successful in stimulating the regeneration of brain cells in laboratory experiments. In contrast to earlier nerve-growth promoting agents, these drugs are made up of small molecules that move freely from the bloodstream into the brain. This ease in movement from bloodstream to brain means that patients would be able to take these drugs by mouth instead of by injection.

So far the effects of neuroimmunophilins in laboratory experiments have been impressive. When animals with a Parkinson-like disease swallow a pill containing the neuroimmunophilin, a 30 percent restoration takes place in the nerve cells within the pathway damaged in Parkinson's disease. This results in functional recovery. In experiments on mice, the addition of a neuroimmunophilin prevents nerve damage and promotes regrowth of already damaged nerve cells. If neuroimmunophilin drugs work as well in humans, it may be possible to reverse some of the effects of Parkinson's disease, which afflicts 2 million people worldwide.

Examples like these make many researchers wonder if pill-induced longevity enhancement could be far behind. Rather than a science fiction scenario, it might prove to be a logical extension of naturally occurring nerve cell preservation and regeneration, according to Burton S. Singer of the Office of Population Research at Princeton University.

Singer points to a study of older women carried out at the University of Wisconsin. Rather than deteriorating with age, these women actually showed improvement in their mental functioning in the years from sixty-five to seventy-five.

"When you look at cognitive improvement studies on the elderly, it is conceivable that there is some generation of new brain cells going on in humans as well. The idea that brain cells never regenerate may not be true in humans. As a result of the neuroimmunophilin work, we know it is not true in mice. And we also know, in mice, that new brain cell development is taking place. So we should not rush to judgment that a similar process isn't taking place in human brains as well," he says.

Inevitably, the idea of building new brain cells raises another question: Why not a total brain transplant?

A brain transplant between two human beings would be an incredibly difficult feat—and an undesirable one as well: Our individual identity is intimately linked with the changes undergone by our brains over our lifetime. Our neurons and their unique synaptic connections make us what we are. If we replace brains, we replace neurons and synapses and, essentially, we end up with different people.

This is equally true if new brain cells result from replacement therapies or drugs. Using these methods, would it be possible to regenerate the same synapses and thus the same personality? Not likely. We become different people as we undergo changes in our brain cells and their interconnections. The synaptic connections now existing in our brain could never be exactly duplicated. Thus adding new cells would mean the forging of new connections and in a way a new identity.

Replacement therapies like neuroimmunophilins are likely, therefore, to be used in selective rather than general ways: additional brain cells implanted in areas of deficiency rather than any kind of general addition of cells to the whole brain. These limited brain grafts may correct for age-related impairments in movement, energy generation, and information processing. But large-scale modifications of personality via brain cell infusions will remain in the realm of science fiction. And isn't that all to the good? No one wants to think of himself or herself requiring a change in identity to stay healthily alive until 100.

CHAPTER 6

Learn to foresee consequences.
Pace yourself.

REMEMBER, IT'S A SMALL WORLD and a long life. The centenarian must learn to think in terms of decades rather than days or weeks. We're the only creatures capable of taking the long view. That's why strategic thinking about what science is discovering is important: to make our tactical actions add up to something. A dog is a tactical thinker; it doesn't see farther into the future than the next opportunity for a meal or the chance to be let out into the yard for a romp. But we have some capacity to foresee the likely consequences of our present actions and learn to plan ahead so we can reap the future rewards stemming from wise decisions made now. It's the frontal lobes of our brain that give us this prescient sense.

Frontal Lobes

Scientists learned about the frontal lobes by observing the consequences of damage in that area. Phineas Gage, a nineteenth-century railroad foreman, sustained a devastating injury to his frontal lobes. Afterward, his personality changed from that of a conscientious, dependable employee to an irascible, unpredictable man who could neither give nor follow directions. It was the frontal lobe damage that wreaked that havoc on Gage's personality. From this sad example, scientists gained their first insight into a basic brain principle: Most of the qualities that set us apart from other animals similar to ourselves depend on normally intact frontal lobes.

In comparison with every other creature on earth, the human brain has dramatically enlarged frontal lobes. Located just behind our forehead, the frontal lobes are a full 200 percent larger in us than in our primate cousins. They are the last cortical areas to mature: their development continues throughout adolescence and into maturity. In addition, the frontal lobes are connected to almost every other part of the brain, including the limbic system, a superhighway of connecting sites that makes it possible for us to experience and express emotion.

Several interesting consequences result from the organization of our frontal lobes. First, we are eminently proactive creatures, capable of taking the initiative and anticipating events. Only we can take the necessary steps now to increase our chances of becoming centenarians. Many of the factors that will make that 100-plus goal possible are already known to us: never smoke, buckle your seatbelts, injury-proof your home, take sensible precautions against potential muggers. Additional proactive steps we can take are discussed in other parts of this book.

The point is that we are not limited to simply reacting to events: We can at every moment take immediate steps to change those things about ourselves that endanger us. Such a view isn't currently popular among those who would convince us that none of us is responsible for our own actions, or that we are all "victims" of one sort of another. But brain research on the frontal lobes supports just the opposite conclusion.

At any given moment normal frontal lobe function provides us with a means of comparing what we are now with what we would like to be. Brain scientists call this "working memory." Let's elaborate on that just a bit:

Imagine yourself for a moment as an executive like David Mahoney, chairing a meeting to draw up the budget for the next year with his top three personnel. One of the three is very conservative and wary. He loads his budget numbers, projecting a need for more money than is probably necessary. He doesn't do this because he is dishonest or incompetent. Rather, he's just trying to protect his division against any shortfalls in available cash.

The second person at the meeting is more confident: She sees the company doing well and generating enough capital over the next few months to counter the need for huge budgetary commitments.

The third person isn't sure and holds no strong opinion about how high or how low the budget should be.

David: "In situations like that I have to think on many levels at once. Take that first person with the strong opinion that things may not go right. I have to find out why he feels that way and try to bring him to a more neutral position. I don't try to change him, at least not by confronting him. Who knows? He might be right and I want to hear him out. I have to ask myself while listening to each of them: Why is he or she coming to this conclusion?

"At Norton Simon, Inc., where I was CEO, I had to make these kinds of decisions all the time. I had to integrate the opinions of my managers: adjust for the tendency of some managers to load their numbers and make them higher with the tendency of other managers to low-ball them. In the final analysis I was the sum total of all of those numbers. I had to reconcile them and come up with my best judgment about what the budget really should be. That judgment then had to be passed on to the board of directors and then to stockholders. At every stage of this process, every observation and thought and hunch had to be evaluated so I could figure out nine months in advance where the company was going to come out. All of these judgments were going on all the time in tandem and in different directions."

Richard: "I've seen David in action during one of these sessions. In addition to the things he mentions above, he was dealing with an inflow of phone calls, e-mail messages, faxes, and, of course, the human distractions of assistants and secretaries coming into the room to remind him of things he must not forget to do later in the day and people he must call after the meeting. Competing with all of this was some classical music playing on a stereo in the background. It takes almost a superhuman effort not to be distracted by all of this information. There are also the internal distractions."

As David conducts the meeting he may find his attention intermittently interrupted by thoughts of other unsolved problems awaiting his attention. Or he may momentarily think of last weekend's football game. While focusing his attention on the meeting, he must maintain a keen appreciation of time. He has to tailor the meeting so it doesn't go on longer than the allotted time. In addition, he has to make sure everybody understands the management decision once the decision is made. He also has to keep in mind the results of the present meeting and balance it with what he hopes to achieve in future meetings.

This example illustrates something that every one of us does every day. Present intentions (the meeting) must be integrated with events in the past and plans for the future. Things must be put into context. Finally, attention has to be focused to prevent the intrusion of external distractions or internal mental activities.

In the example of David's meeting, he has to hold online, to borrow a computer term, events from the past and present while linking them with the future. All of these processes are carried out by our frontal lobes. How do we know this?

Brain scientists have observed for more than 100 years that people with damaged frontal lobes lose their ability to do all of the seemingly simple processes involved in the meeting example. Time-locked in the present and lacking the ability to anticipate the future or link with the past, the frontally injured person lacks personal continuity. He or she just drifts from one thing to another without a sense of purpose. Obviously, long-term planning is impossible under such circumstances.

Our normally functioning frontal lobes perform five major functions for us:

First, they provide the underpinning for our drives and motivation. We know this because in cases of frontal lobe damage the person is listless and apathetic; such a person does nothing unless somebody forces him or her.

Second, the frontal lobes help us get the Big Picture by sequencing and linking bits of information into meaningful wholes, such as earnings per share and cash flow, or the rate of inflation and what it will cost to send one's kids to college.

Third, the frontal lobes are responsible for probably the most important exercise of the human mind, executive control: planning and anticipating the consequences of behavior. It is this function that is most important in self-pacing.

Almost without exception, the really worthwhile things in life require us to postpone present satisfaction for the sake of greater satisfaction later. You don't become a brain surgeon overnight. Before being certified to perform that first solo operation on the brain, you have to put in six or more years after medical school. It's the frontal lobes that enable you to get through the grind by allowing you to see beyond present inconvenience and hassle and continue applied efforts toward the attainment of your goals.

Fourth, and closely related to the third function, is "future memory." This involves building up a model in your mind of your goals and using that internal model of the future as a guide for altering and updating your behavior toward goal achievement.

Finally, the frontal lobes provide us with that important sense of continuity so necessary to avoid repetitive changes of mind about what we want and what we are willing to do to get it. Those of us with intact and normally functioning frontal lobes are capable of enhancing our frontal lobe powers. Indeed, that is exactly what we are suggesting when we suggest that you pace yourself and keep your sights on the long haul.

Many of us are already doing just that in one area of our lives: weight control. Everyone who has ever been on a diet knows that the hardest part of weight loss is keeping the weight off. Yet this difficulty doesn't stem from ignorance; we know full well how we can maintain our hard-fought weight loss: Keep doing whatever we did to lose weight in the first place. The difficulty comes from not sticking with the diets and weight loss programs. Successful and sustained weight loss demands constant attention to diet and lifestyle. A person who wishes to remain slim uses his or her frontal lobes constantly. All five major frontal lobe functions mentioned above must be called into play. It's those frontal lobes that make sustained dedication possible.

Similar lifetime dedication is needed to live to be 100. Through enhanced frontal lobe functioning we can persist in the efforts needed to increase our chances of becoming healthy centenarians. That phrase "increase our chances" is an important one. There are no guarantees about longevity, no matter how healthily we live or how well we take care of ourselves. But even though most of us won't live to be 100, our efforts to achieve and maintain a healthier lifestyle will carry their own reward: All of us will feel better and likely suffer less pain and disability.

Even if we individually don't make it to 100, our children and grandchildren have a good shot at it. Our children and grandchildren have the advantage of a large amount of knowledge available to them about healthy living. They're also savvy about the perils that must be avoided. It's this knowledge, much of it based on science, particularly neuroscience, that gives them the decisive edge over older folks who may have practiced some bad health habits earlier in life.

The key is to take the long view, and since the long view is made up of a lot of short views, it's important to everything you do almost daily. Use those frontal lobes.

CHAPTER 7

Use it or lose It. Take active measures now to combat disuse atrophy.

CERTAIN CELLS IN AREAS OF THE BRAIN beneath the cortex (called subcortical nuclei) are sometimes irreverently dubbed the "juice machines." They give us enthusiasm and general "get up and go" energy. When Samuel Johnson said, "The question is not so much 'Is it worth seeing?' but rather, 'Is it worth going to see?'" he was unknowingly referring to the subcortical nuclei, which generate enthusiasm and energy.

With aging, almost everyone undergoes some loss of cells in the subcortical nuclei. It's what we notice when we joke that our get-up-and-go "got up and went." Since this is natural, our task is to recognize that we are "mellowing" rather than losing any of our abilities. Our attention to those abilities, as intact as ever, helps us maintain mental vigor.

Every talent and special skill that you've developed over your lifetime is represented in your brain by a complex network of neurons. And each time you engage in any activity that involves your talents and skills, the neuronal linkages in that network are enhanced. Think of the brain cells as shaped like trees composed of long branches subdividing into smaller and smaller branches. As the result of brain growth and the person's experience in the world, tremendous overlap and connectivity develop among the tree branches. Neuroscientists, struck with the tree analogy, refer to this process as "arborization."

Eventually nerve cells form active circuits based on these branchlike linkages. The more often the circuits are activated, the easier it is to activate them the next time. Subjectively, you experience this as the formation of a habit. With time the activity gets easier to do; the more the skill or talent is practiced, the better you get at it. But if you neglect your talents and skills, they begin to wane, and over time it becomes harder and harder to perform at your best. If enough time passes you will experience great difficulty returning to your former level of excellence. That's because the neuronal circuits have fallen into disuse: greater degrees of effort are required to activate them. But no matter how long you've neglected a skill, you'll never find yourself in the same situation as the person who never learned the skill in the first place.

Neuronal circuits, once established, never entirely disappear. It's the ease of facilitating them that varies. This law of facilitation and disuse atrophy applies to every activity, whether physical or mental. Neglect your tennis or your golf for enough time and your skills in these very different activities will deteriorate.

Remember that the brain is an ever-changing organ. If one part gets rusty and suffers atrophy from disuse, its functions are taken over by other areas that are used more. When we stop challenging ourselves and expanding, or at least maintaining our skills, the brain cells involved in the neuronal networks drop out and link into other networks. Eventually the skill has almost entirely disappeared. We say *almost* because some neurons, though a much smaller number, always remain in the network.

If you haven't bowled in twenty years, then your initial scores are going to be predictably low. But you will still do better than someone who has never bowled. That's because some of the neurons from that circuit you established years ago are still functioning in a simpler, less elaborated network. As a result, we never entirely lose a talent we have once developed. The key point: Practice enough to keep all of the neurons active in those networks you wish to maintain. Obviously, as we change over the years, certain activities lose their interest for us. As a child, Richard was skilled at marbles and, later, pool, two activities he no longer engages in. As a result, the neuronal networks underlying these childhood and adolescent interests are no longer highly facilitated. His skill levels in these activities have dropped accordingly. What's important is picking and choosing what skills and activities you want to keep current.

Scientists believe that by using what you don't want to lose for a half hour two to three times a week you won't get rusty and you'll maintain your skills and talents. At middle age and beyond, the greatest benefit comes from small, consistently applied efforts. By practicing skills even just a little each week those skills can be maintained, even expanded. Here are some rules for how to do that:

- Be consistent in your practice routines. Try to practice at the same time each day so the brain will be primed and ready to get the maximum out of each session.

- Keep challenging yourself. Throw away your calculator and get back into the habit of adding things up yourself. When you get your daily newspaper, make up your own mind about the meaning of the events reported on the first page before turning to the editorial pages. In that way you've thought things through for yourself and haven't just gone along with somebody else's ideas.

- Try to avoid inner and outer criticisms. Each of us has incorporated an inner critic—sometimes the voice of an overly demanding parent or early boss who tells us we aren't doing well enough. When you become aware of those critics calling to you from your past, silence them if they have no case.

- Keep in mind the role models that attracted you to the activity in the first place. He or she may have been a patient, kindly coach or instructor who went over the fundamentals again and again until you finally "got it." *Become* that teacher.

- Don't fall into the "pro trap." Many people become discouraged because they cannot imagine themselves performing at the high levels exemplified by the professionals. While admiring the performance of the very best in the field, remind yourself that your goals are different: to keep your abilities alive, not to become a champion.

Think of the brain as a dynamic, ever-changing organ linked to the rest of the body through the powerful brain-body interaction. Moreover, scientists now are certain of our ability to wittingly or unwittingly affect this interaction through conscious actions and decisions. This ability for us to control our own health and destiny has great consequences when it comes to our next topic: stress.

CHAPTER 8

Learn to handle stress. Your brain alertness and longevity are going to depend on how well you handle stress.

EACH OF US IS ENGAGED in an elaborate juggling game involving work, family, intimate relationships, and self-interest. And managing these separate, interrelated areas of our lives creates stress.

Contrary to popular opinion, stress is not just another term for tension or pressure. Nor is stress always unhealthy. "One man's stress is another man's challenge" is a better way of thinking about it. Public speaking, for instance, is something both of us enjoy; but we also know many people for whom standing up and speaking in public ranks right up there with skydiving with a parachute that can't be guaranteed to open.

Stress is best thought of as the way we respond to a physical or emotional demand. That demand may be something as unpleasant as the notification of a tax audit or as exciting as learning you've just won the lottery. In many instances stress is internally defined. David recalls the stress experienced at Officers' Candidate School at Fort Benning, Georgia:

"We all had to take what they called confidence courses. One day you would be climbing cargo nets hand over hand. The next day you would have to walk along two-by-fours at increasing heights. It was the same task at twenty feet above the ground as it was with the two-by-fours flat on the ground. But the result wasn't the same. Some guys choked at the greater height. They had to learn how to handle stress. They did this by convincing themselves that the task was the same at whatever height. They had to mentally transform the experience in such a way that it was no longer stressful. Today that kind of training forms the basis of programs such as Outward Bound. Young people learn through wilderness experience that stress is internally determined. They learn how to transform stress into challenge. In that way they feel more confident about themselves, their self-esteem rises, and they live longer, healthier lives."

Neuroscientists are now convinced that people who overreact to stress lead shorter lives and are more susceptible to accelerated brain and nervous system disease. In animals this hyperreactivity is genetic, and the individual animal can't do much about it. But we humans can change the terms by reinterpreting the situation. That's because, as some forward-thinking physicians have been telling us for the past fifteen years, the brain and the body are one.

When your brain is healthy, your body does a better job of resisting illness. When your body is functioning at its best, your feelings are more positive. That's why understanding how stress works on your physical and mental health can help you to manage that stress better and live longer.

To Robert M. Sapolsky, professor of biological sciences and neuroscience at Stanford University, stress-related diseases represent inappropriate and maladaptive bodily responses:

"A large body of evidence suggests that stress-related disease emerges, predominantly, out of the fact that we so often activate a physiological system that has evolved for responding to physical emergencies, but we turn it on for months on end, worrying about mortgages, relationships, and promotions."

As Sapolsky makes clear in his book *Why Zebras Don't Get Ulcers*, "We humans can be stressed by things that simply make no sense to zebras. It is not a general mammalian trait to become anxious about mortgages, or the Internal Revenue Service, about public speaking or what you will say in a job interview, about the inevitability of death."

Rather than stress resulting from physical threats to our health and safety, ". . . our human experience is replete with psychological stressors, a far cry from the physical world of hunger, injury, blood loss, or temperature extremes."

The physiological system that gives us our capacity to activate stress is called the autonomic nervous system. This is a network of nerves that project from the brain, down the spine and out to the smooth muscles and glands of our internal organs, to the skin, and to the blood vessels. The nerves projecting to these areas carry messages that are relatively involuntary and automatic, hence the name autonomic nervous system.

For instance, the stomach "grumbling" that you hear and experience when you haven't eaten for a long time occurs because of activation of nerve fibers within the lining of the intestinal tract. Such activation occurs "automatically," outside of your conscious control, and even despite your embarrassed efforts to quiet the rumbling.

The autonomic nervous system consists of two divisions: the sympathetic and the parasympathetic. The half of the autonomic nervous system that activates the body toward maximal exertion (the "fight or flight" reaction) is the sympathetic nervous system. It's that part of the autonomic nervous system that prepares the body to handle life-and-death situations.

If while walking down a dark street at night you hear light

footsteps rapidly approaching from behind, your heart and breathing rates will increase, your muscles will tense in anticipation of running, and the hairs on your skin will literally "stand up" (secondary to the contraction of tiny muscles attaching the hairs to the skin surface). Increased amounts of glucose are made available for use by your leg muscles. Activating hormones are secreted by the brain and the adrenal glands. Acting in concert, all of these changes brought about by the sympathetic nervous system prepare you for handling the emergency.

Opposed to the action of the sympathetic nervous system is a set of nerves that are responsible for bringing about and maintaining states of calm and tranquillity. When you sit back and "relax" after a good meal, think pleasant thoughts, and generally experience the world in a calm and collected frame of mind, your parasympathetic nervous system is in play. At such times you're experiencing what psychologists often refer to as the "relaxation response." Your heart is beating more slowly and less forcefully; your lungs are expanding and contracting fewer times per minute; your brain and endocrine glands are no longer spewing out stimulating or exciting hormones.

Stress results from an overreaction of the sympathetic nervous system under inappropriate circumstances. Running from that stranger encountered in the dark alley is an appropriate response made possible by the firing up of the sympathetic nervous system. But if your sympathetic nervous system fires up every time the boss walks into your office, the response is not appropriate (at least we hope not). In such instances you're the victim of a debilitating stress response. Moreover, this stress response can be fatal.

A patient who enters surgery in a state of stressful foreboding is more likely to suffer some type of operative complication, according to studies carried out at Johns Hopkins Medical Center. The better your mental state going into the surgery—the less stressed you feel about the outcome—the better you're going to do.

Heart attacks, ulcers, migraine headaches, irritable bowel symptoms—these are only some of the consequences of stress-induced illness resulting from a habitually overreactive sympathetic nervous system.

While most of the stress research has involved physical stress such as heart attacks, seizures, and tumors, mental stress is believed to be just as harmful. Certainly animal studies point in this direction. (Obviously an animal can't tell you what it finds stressful or when it is feeling stressed.)

A mouse that hears a warning buzzer seconds before receiving an electric shock (a stressful event for any creature, we can reasonably infer) gets fewer ulcers than a mouse deprived of the warning buzzer. Stress is also influenced by a sense of control. Give the animal a lever that, when pushed, terminates the shock, and ulcers are cut way down. This even works under test conditions when the lever is completely disconnected from the shock apparatus. It's not the actual control that matters as much as the animal's belief that it has control.

As a result of research such as this carried out on animals, we have a new understanding of the harmful effects of stress in ourselves. We now know that mental events exert harmful effects on the brain and are transmitted to the body. This knowledge has spurred the evolution of effective techniques and principles aimed at lowering or avoiding stress. It's called stress management.

Predictability and control determine whether we experience stress or how much stress we experience. For example, loud noises are not nearly as stressful under circumstances when something can be done to stop them. The shouting and screaming from the kids in the yard next door will stress you more than similar noise from your own kids: you have some control (probably limited) over your own kids, but can't, realistically, exert any dependable influence on the decibel level prevailing in your neighbor's yard.

In one example of the importance of control, a Duke University psychiatric study looked at 152 women employees in the customer service and paperwork-processing department of a large corporation. The psychiatrists found heightened stress responses among women who were required ". . . to complete a great deal of work in too short a period and also on jobs in which employees do a lot of repetitive work while not being allowed to make decisions on their own, to learn new skills, or to develop special abilities."

But stress can also come from the neurotic need for too much control. David encountered this about two weeks before the 1968 presidential election.

After a full day of campaigning, Richard Nixon was relaxing in his hotel suite at the Waldorf-Astoria. "We were all talking in different groups," recalls David. " At one point Nixon waved me to the back room and said, 'David, you're a New Yorker. Do you know a place we can go and listen to some piano music? Sneak out of here and I will see you in the hall.' I then went ahead and called Goldie's, a prominent piano/jazz bar at the time.

"To my surprise Goldie alerted the audience that Nixon was coming, and when we arrived the audience broke out into applause. After about an hour of music the captain came over to me and told me there was a phone call for me. Without batting an eye, Nixon said, 'It is undoubtedly Haldeman.' He was right.

"On the phone I encountered the angry suggestion that I must be 'out of [my] mind' to take Nixon to such a place just days before the election. I never did have a good answer other than one that would have probably angered him even more: The future president was enjoying that brief respite, and maybe even picked up a few votes.

"Maybe Haldeman would have met a nicer end later if he had been more relaxed and less stressed."

Job stress leads to increased anxiety and anger, reduced social support, and negative feelings toward coworkers and supervisors, according to the Duke University psychiatrists. All of these factors are known to increase the likelihood of heart attacks and death.

Social Support

Do you know what is the greatest protection against the harmful effects of stress? It's other people. If you have a friend or somebody you can count on, it makes all the difference in the world.

David says: "After my open-heart surgery to repair a mitral valve, I can still remember how good I felt and what a help it was to me to open my eyes in the recovery room and see at the foot of my bed my three best friends in the world. my wife, Hillie, my son David, and my lifetime best pal, the writer Bill Safire. The feeling of stress just washed out of me at that moment. And I'm convinced their presence made a difference in my recovery."

Nor is that just David and Richard's opinion. In one study of patients suffering from coronary artery disease, half of those without friends and relatives were dead within five years—a rate three times higher than among patients with spouses or friends.

Social support—in plain words, friends and relatives—can protect people in stress from a wide variety of physical and mental hazards. This can include low-birth-weight infants, arthritis, tuberculosis, depression, alcoholism, family breakdown, and death. Further, friends and family can reduce the amount of medication required to treat illnesses, accelerate recovery, and increase compliance with doctors' orders.

Without friends you can count on during times of stress, you start depending too much on crutches such as alcohol, tobacco, or tranquilizers. In a study of university students during exam time, smoking increased by an average of 54 percent in women who had few friends. But alcohol intake decreased 17.5 percent among students spending time with friends; the "loners," in contrast, increased their drinking by almost 20 percent.

Highly emotional people are especially susceptible to stress. Those who score high on emotionality, when compared to calmer, less emotional people, report more hassles. The highly emotional people also show more symptoms under stress than do other people who are lower on the emotionality scale. In short, if you tend to "blow a fuse" when faced with frustration, you're not only going to experience more stress, you're also likely to die earlier from stress-related illnesses.

Information Overload

Technology provides a new source of stress: information overload. Many of us read a daily newspaper (and many people read more than one) and tune in to news broadcasts. Did you know that the daily *New York Times* contains more information than the average person in the seventeenth century encountered over a lifetime? Think about the adjustment that such an increase in information intake demands of the human brain.

As an added stress, much of the news is inherently disturbing: serial killers roaming the country, crack-addicted mothers abusing and even murdering their children, drive-by shootings in our major cities, the constant conflict between the sexes and across generations. As TV producers say, "If it bleeds, it leads."

Cultural and media experts may disagree whether this flood of negative information is reflective of how our society actually is, or whether the news is being shaped according to what

Richard once dubbed at a Smithsonian International Symposium as "media Darwinism": the survival of the starkest, the most intensely stimulating, the most extreme, the most revolting, and so on.

But whatever the cause, the news has become so stressful that many mental health experts such as Andrew Weil in his *Eight Weeks to Optimum Health* advocate not reading or watching any news at all. Since both of us are confirmed news junkies, we don't go that far. But the brain is adept at handling only so much information per unit of time. Beyond this, additional information only leads to additional stress. Moreover, much of the information that is seemingly inseparable from our day-to-day lives is unnecessary or irrelevant.

Take the weather reports on television, for instance. How much do you need to know about the weather to determine how to dress or whether it would make sense to take along an umbrella? Yet who hasn't spent ten or fifteen minutes watching the local weather person explaining details of tomorrow's weather that are comprehensible only to a meteorologist?

Unless you're a doctor or someone likely to become involved in life-or-death situations, do you really need a pager, a cell phone, and a laptop computer during your weekend at the beach? Granted, many of these technological information gatherers and dispensers serve the purpose of ego massage. It's nice to feel important, and who doesn't need on occasion to bolster one's own ego by impressing others? But such perks can carry a higher price than simply their cost. Impatience, the feeling of being chronically overloaded, jitteriness, burnout, overindulgence in alcohol—these are some of the costs exacted if you don't control information technology rather than letting it control you.

Loss of control over a deluge of information is wreaking havoc in the corporate world, according to a study by the

Institute for the Future, a consulting firm based in Menlo Park, California. "Today's corporate staff are inundated with so many communication tools—fax, electronic mail, teleconferencing, postal mail, interoffice mail, voice mail, and others—that sometimes they don't know which to turn to for even the simplest tasks," according to the Institute report for Pitney-Bowes.

Stress results from the sheer volume of information: The average worker sends and receives 178 messages every day. The result is a frustrating and predictable vicious circle. In self-defense against information overload, workers begin to cut themselves off from the stream whenever possible; voice mails and e-mails are ignored, lengthy faxes left unread, postal mail left unattended on the desk. But this attempt at self-insulation only compounds the problem, since others are doing the same thing. Stress and frustration escalate as each information-over-burdened worker tries harder and harder to stand out from the mountain of information inundating other workers. Thus the same message may be faxed, e-mailed, and voice-recorded again and again to increase the likelihood of getting the message through.

No one is claiming, incidentally, that we would be better off without these information-gathering and information-disseminating tools. Rather, we are suggesting that to avoid stress, we must control them rather than allow them to control us.

Perhaps all of us should take our cues from successful agers. Jeanne Calment, who at 122 reached the oldest authenticated age of any human being in history, lived so long because of her "unflappability." According to her biographer Jean-Marie Robine, "I think she was someone who, constitutionally and biologically speaking, was immune to stress. She once said, 'If you can't do anything about it, don't worry about it.'"

Other successful agers tend to resemble Jeanne Calment. When stressed, they typically rely less on hostile reactions and escapist fantasy regardless of the type of stress. This resistance to stress in later life is especially notable, since neuroscientists have found in their research that age is typically associated with a *lessened* tolerance for stress. Indeed, unhealthy aging can be defined in terms of age-related breakdowns in the management of stress.

Healthy aging, in contrast, is accompanied by a feeling of being in control, rather than at the mercy, of stressful circumstances. Feeling in control is an internal trait that can be learned—just like its opposite, helplessness.

The opposite of feeling stressed is a feeling of well-being. According to Leonard Poon, the director of the University of Georgia's centenarian study, low tension and high extroversion—in essence, social involvement—results in high morale among centenarians.

"They tend not to internally generate stress because they do not take personally life's inevitable frustrations. As they have learned, change is a part of life, and they have come to accept it. The take-home message: If you can't accept change—sometimes change that at least temporarily seems for the worse—you'll never see 100."

How to Reduce Stress

At this point, pause and consider: How do I handle stressors? As a loss of control? A punishment? How can we manage stress and maintain healthy functioning?

Let's remember that juggling act we mentioned at the beginning of this chapter. It's no longer sufficient to do well in two or three of those four areas (work, family, relationships, and self-interest); we have to master all four of them. Author and clinical psychologist Wayne M. Sotile believes that stress results when we concentrate on one area—usually work—and ignore the other three. We don't allow enough time for simple pleasures, thus foregoing the key to managing stress: "resiliency—the ability to recover strength, spirit, and good humor quickly."

Sotile has identified a behavioral pattern he calls "hurry sickness," from which far too many of us suffer. Someone afflicted with "hurry sickness" experiences a prevailing sense of time urgency—there is never enough time to get things done. This leads to impatience with self and others; perfectionism, multitasking (doing too many things at one time), irritability, and temper tantrums when things don't come together as quickly or as easily as anticipated. Sufferers from "hurry sickness" are also competitive with others, controlling, hostile, cynical, and, most characteristic, totally involved in their work.

As an antidote to the stress of "hurry sickness" Sotile suggests we put our best efforts into maintaining our relationships. We need:

- *Tangible support:* someone to help us if we are sick or temporarily disabled.

- *Affectionate support:* someone to show love and affection, make us feel wanted.

- *Positive social interaction:* someone to have a good time with, get together with, and relax with.

- *Emotional/informational support:* someone to listen when we need to talk, give advice in times of crises.

Most people give and receive these supports in a marriage —one of the reasons we advise, later in this book, investing in your family dimension. A happy marriage is associated with a decreased incidence of psychiatric illness, alcohol abuse, suicide, risk of death, and level of stress.

Other time-proven methods of reducing stress include:

1. Learn to "let go" of things that are outside of your control. Numerous studies on managing stress emphasize

the importance of "accepting a stressful situation." That doesn't mean lying down and playing dead. It means you act like a boxer: You accept the challenge, don't give in to panic, put out your best shots, and stop worrying. If you're in over your head this time, there will be other fights in your future.

2. Learn to act when what you do can make a difference.

3. Balance work and recreation. And as will be mentioned in chapter 17, diversify your career from the beginning by taking up a serious avocation.

4. Work off the sense of stress by physical activity. A punching bag is a great means of keeping in shape and expressing hostility in a healthy way.

5. Take frequent breaks during the day. Not only does this create a change of pace, it also often leads to new outlooks or new attitudes.

6. Make yourself available to other people. When bored or lonely, call a friend and do something together. The best way of keeping ourselves in good repair is by tending and nourishing our relationships with others.

7. As a corollary, don't jeopardize your close relationships by talking too much about yourself and your problems. Nobody wants to spend time with a "flooder"—someone who gushes from every pore with highly emotional and upsetting personal feelings and experiences. If you have an irresistible need to talk about your unhappy childhood or how shabbily you are being treated at your office, spare your friends these recitations. If your communications relate to matters concerning your mental health, then spend the necessary money and time on a psychiatrist or other mental health professional.

Take the advice of Hillie Mahoney, David's wife: "Don't use your friends as therapists; in most cases, they are not professionally trained, and you'll only frustrate and confuse them. Negative emotions and their expression should be employed sparingly, because negative thoughts beget negative thoughts. Don't feel you have to talk about them to others, except perhaps to professionals. This isn't being superficial; it's just a recognition that we all have problems and we best help each other by not burdening each other with our individual problems."

8. Get out of yourself by doing something for others. Most of us spend too much time inside our own heads. When we give our time to a person or a cause we believe in, stress disappears. It's amazing how difficult it is to put into practice this oldest and hardest rule: Only by giving do we receive. We will say more about this in chapter 19.

9. Avoid the use of chemicals or food to alter your moods. Avoid sedatives and tranquilizers, limit caffeine, fats, sugar, and alcohol, and never smoke cigarettes.

10. Try to stay in tune with your moods and inner states. If your head aches or your stomach is churning, stop and try to figure out the stressor. If anxious or depressed, don't waste time denying your feelings. Do something physical as an antidote. At such times also move toward, not away from, other people.

11. Finally, when you're under stress, one of the best ways to stop the stress is to breathe slowly and deeply. Rapid, shallow breathing assisted our prehistoric ancestors to prepare for fighting or running. By a curious feedback,

shallow, rapid breathing now induces in the brain all of the mental accompaniments of our ancestors' anxious preparedness: uncomfortable states ranging from a vague feeling of uneasiness to outright terror. You can stop this progression anywhere in its course by breathing just the opposite to the way you breathe when under stress. Start by breathing in through the nose. Count silently to 5 as the lower abdomen fills with air and expands outward (not just the expansion of the chest—the hallmark of shallow breathing). Then expel the air slowly through your mouth during another silent count to 5. Do this for two minutes or more.

Of course, some of life's experiences are inherently stressful and involve powerful negative emotions that cannot be avoided. Being told you have cancer, for instance, is going to be stressful no matter what your attitude. And we're certainly not selling the view that all of life's problems can be managed simply by adopting stress reduction techniques. Rather, we are suggesting that stress reduction is more of a health enhancing life orientation than simply a hodgepodge of gimmicks and techniques.

Your chances of becoming a centenarian or of living a long and healthy life to whatever age depend on how successfully you manage stress in your daily life. Perhaps no area of brain-body interaction is as important as this, and perhaps no other is so much within your ability to influence.

CHAPTER 9

Develop an optimistic attitude toward life. Optimists not only live better, they also live longer.

TO SUPPORT YOUR LONGEVITY, optimism is a longer-range proposition. Unlike stress managment, your optimism should be nonreactive and, at its best, pretty near impenetrable by outside influence. It should be as resistant to collapse as the posts and studs of a well-built house. And best of all, like a house, it can be built.

Optimism protects against depression, and depression can kill. Most illnesses, especially things such as headaches, backaches, high blood pressure, and heart disease, can be caused or at least influenced by our feelings.

The Johns Hopkins School of Hygiene and Public Health studied this issue in a group of patients over a fourteen-year period and found that depressed individuals are four times more likely to suffer a heart attack than their optimistic, nondepressed counterparts. According to William W. Eaten, the director of the study, depression is as much of a risk factor for heart disease as elevated levels of cholesterol.

Just as peace is more than the absence of war, so optimism

is far more than just the absence of depression. Psychiatrists rightly insist that depression is a disease. But physicians and laymen alike agree that optimism exerts a protective effect against the development of depression: you cannot be both optimistic and depressed.

People who have heart disease and in addition suffer from depression die at a much higher rate than patients with only heart disease do. One school of thought believes that heart disease results from a series of biochemical changes in depressed people. Their hearts beat faster, adjust less efficiently to changes in activity level, and pump blood throughout the body at a higher level of blood pressure. Stress hormones are also increased, which leads to disturbances in heart rate and rhythm. Finally, depressed people have a harder time motivating themselves to enhance their physical and mental fitness. Lacking the energy and enthusiasm that accompanies optimism, the depressed person doesn't exercise and fails to comply with medication programs. He or she is also more likely to abuse alcohol, tobacco, or drugs to provide a temporary lift in spirits.

Optimism about the general state of one's health has a measurable impact on mortality. A negative evaluation of one's health is associated with increased mortality in studies of men in Europe and Japan. The answers to two questions—"What do you think of your health compared to other men of your age?" and "How would you assess your own health?"—served as indicators of early mortality. Those men with optimistic positive responses to these questions lived longer than those who expressed doubts about their health.

But what about people in bad health who have good reason for negative expressions about the state of their health ("poor-health realists")? Even here an optimistic attitude, "health optimism," conferred longevity benefits. "While poor-health realists were at the highest risk of dying within a three-year period, health optimists were significantly less likely to die than poor-health realists, in spite of sharing similar health status," according to a study from Case Western Reserve University titled "The Meaning of Older Adults' Health Appraisals."

In addition to optimism's influence on health in the short run, positive self-ratings about health—in essence, optimism about one's health—serve as an independent predictor of longevity. This is true irrespective of a person's actual objective state of health as assessed by a doctor. Optimism about your health, in other words, exerts a measurable influence on what level of health you are likely to experience and how long you are likely to live.

Maintaining an optimistic attitude can also speed up recovery when you are sick, according to Michael Scheier, a psychologist at Carnegie Mellon University in Pittsburgh. Dispositional optimism, as Scheier calls it, is a relatively stable, generalized expectation that good outcomes will occur across important life domains. He has even come up with a ten-question life orientation test that measures a person's tendency for optimism over pessimism.

Pause here for a moment to answer the ten questions:

___ 1. In uncertain times, I usually expect the best.
___ 2. It's easy for me to relax.
___ 3. If something can go wrong for me, it will.
___ 4. I'm always optimistic about my future.
___ 5. I enjoy my friends a lot.
___ 6. It's important for me to keep busy.
___ 7. I hardly ever expect things to go my way.
___ 8. I don't get upset too easily.
___ 9. I rarely count on good things happening to me.
___ 10. Overall, I expect more good things to happen to me than bad.

Score on the following basis:

0 = strongly disagree

1 = disagree

2 = neutral

3 = agree

4 = strongly agree

To arrive at your score you'll need to apply to questions 3, 7, and 9 what psychologists refer to as reverse coding. This makes up for the tendency we all have to cheat just a little bit by putting our best foot forward. For those questions, make the following conversions: 0=4, 1=3, 3=1, and 4=0.

In other words, if you scored 4 (strongly agree) for question 3, change it to 0 (strongly disagree). And do the same reverse coding for questions 7 and 9. Once this is done, total your score only for questions 1, 3, 4, 7, 9, and 10. Questions 2, 5, 6 and 8 are just distracters put in to disguise the true purpose of the test, measuring optimism.

The results are plotted along the following scale in percentages from most pessimistic to most optimistic: 0–12 (0–25%); 13–15 (25–50%); 16–17 (50–75%); and 18–24 (75–100%). Thus, if you scored 19, you are among the top 25 percent of optimistic people.

Scheier has discovered that the greater a person's sense of optimism, the greater his or her ability to successfully cope with stress and hardship. His findings on heart disease agree with the research at Johns Hopkins. For instance, among men undergoing coronary bypass operations, the optimists recover more quickly, often walking earlier and earning increased estimations of functional recovery from hospital staff members. At six months the optimists express greater life satisfaction; have resumed most of their prior activities; and are much less likely, compared with their pessimistic counterparts, to have suffered a heart attack. At the end of five years the optimists are more likely to be working full time, sleeping more soundly, and expressing satisfaction with their health.

Optimism exerts an influence on mortality even among people with the same health status. Those who view their situation less critically ("I'm doing about as well as one could expect under the circumstances") tend to do better than those who concentrate on what they can no longer do. This is particularly true among older people.

One study, from Canada, even concluded that the interplay of optimism and health in older patients might argue for changing the way they are treated by doctors. "The practical implication is that perhaps more attention should be focused on efforts to improve older people's satisfaction with their life situation rather than on marginal improvements of their medical condition."

Do optimists do anything different from pessimists that might explain these results? Here are the various coping strategies that Scheier found among optimists and pessimists. The first nine of the coping strategies tend to be used by optimists, while the tenth through the fourteenth characterize pessimists.

1. Active coping: taking action, exerting efforts, to remove stressors.

2. Planning: thinking about how to confront the stressor, planning one's active coping efforts.

3. Seeking instrumental social support: seeking assistance, information, or advice about what to do.

4. Seeking emotional social support: getting sympathy or emotional support from someone.

5. Suppression of competing activities: concentrating on dealing with the stressor.

6. Religion: increased involvement with religious activities.

7. Positive reinterpretation and growth: making the best of the situation by growing from it or viewing it in a more favorable light.

8. Restraint coping: holding back one's coping attempts to the optimal time.

9. Acceptance: accepting the fact that a stressful event has occurred and is real.

10. Focus on and venting of emotions: an increased awareness of one's emotional distress, and an accompanying tendency to ventilate or discharge those feelings.

11. Denial: rejection of the reality of the stressful event.

12. Mental disengagement: psychological disengagement through daydreaming, sleep, or self-distraction.

13. Behavioral disengagement: giving up or withdrawing.

14. Alcohol/drug use: using chemicals to cope.

15. Humor: making jokes about the stressor.

Humor, the last strategy, can be used by either pessimists (primarily black humor) or by optimists (the jokes tend to be less grim and less cynical). In general, optimists tend to be problem-focused rather than emotionally focused. A problem focuser believes that stressful and life-threatening events such as illnesses can be changed for the better.

The bottom line: Optimists enjoy life more and experience less distress in bad times because they employ healthier, more adaptive coping strategies. Because they are confident and hopeful, they do not disengage from problems, stop trying, or become depressed, but instead they refocus on their life goals and activities. When this is impossible they change these goals according to circumstantial demands.

We're not pushing a Pollyannaish approach to hard times. We all sometimes make business and personal mistakes that no amount of optimism can overcome. In such instances, tactical withdrawal—a temporary "blue funk"—may be the best course to follow, accompanied soon by optimism that in the bigger picture, things will work out. Believe us: in the long run, optimism really does get results. It's the timing that counts. As Kenny Rogers sings it in "The Gambler," you have to "know when to hold 'em, know when to fold 'em."

Optimism also conforms to wisdom extending back many centuries. If you think optimistically, you become imbued with optimism. "All that we are is the result of what we have thought" is a truth that can be traced at least as far back as the Dhamapadda. An Irish aphorism holds that "A man becomes the song he sings." Most exciting of all, optimism is a learnable personality trait.

We can remake ourselves into optimists if we want to badly enough and try hard enough. We hear a lot these days about reinventing ourselves. There's no better more healthful reinvention than to induce optimism until it becomes second nature.

As a first step, force the attitude of optimism, pretending it, making yourself speak and act optimistically. This optimistic behavior, if continued long enough and forcefully enough, often leads to a feeling of optimism. The persona becomes the person.

Don't think of yourself as a "phony" when you pretend something you don't feel. Attitude is probably the most important motivating factor in our lives. If it's good, the world is our oyster; if it's bad, if we sell ourselves short, the game is already lost. Remember: We can induce feelings in ourselves by acting like the feelings already exist. This acting isn't hypocrisy; it's just good mental health.

It's also supported by recent brain findings: Imaging scientists at Washington University in St. Louis proved that the healthy brain will take your commands about how to feel. The researchers rounded up a group of healthy young adults, put them in a PET scanner, and asked them to think of things that would make them feel sad. The volunteers' brain activity during the sad tasks was strikingly similar to that of patients suffering from clinical depression, except in the volunteers the brain activation had been self-induced. That's why, when cognitive therapy studies report improvements in depressed patients, many hard-boiled neuroscientists believe them, whereas they might have been skeptical a few years ago. Such findings also give credibility to a slogan of another group—Alcoholics Anonymous—whose members often tell newcomers skeptical of being happy in sobriety, "Fake it till you make it."

Another way of putting it: Don't dwell on the negative. Nobel laureate and neuroscientist Francis Crick has a sign on his desk with these words: "I'm an old man and I've seen many problems. Most of them never happened." Most of us can't even remember the things that were worrying us ten years ago. Somehow or other, things worked out.

This is one of the reasons why we can't think of depression as purely chemical. It's true that neuroscientists are now working on the biochemical basis of depression, but for centuries people had some success in warding off depression by means of an optimistic mental attitude. "This, too, shall pass" is a motto of the optimist. Of course, part of the problem we have in remaining optimistic stems from our difficulty with trust. We have trouble trusting. Yet we don't have any choice but to trust that things are going to work out. When we're in an airplane, we have to trust that the pilot knows what he or she is doing. Not all decisions are for us to make.

Lack of trust has great mental health consequences. One of the characteristics of the neurotic personality is difficulty with trustful optimism. Everything is always vaguely ominous or threatening. Treatment often involves encouraging the patient not to take on a lot of unnecessary burdens for things he or she can do nothing about.

Other practical steps to encourage optimism include:

Find a role model. Observe and learn from a person who tries to make the best of every situation. Find out by observing and even asking how he or she maintains optimistic behavior. Then try to do what that person does. Don't worry about originality here. There are times when following must come before leading. Building up an optimistic lifestyle is one of them.

Secondly, pay careful attention to the things you tell yourself. Psychologists call this "self-talk" and remaining aware of it is perhaps the most critical aspect of maintaining optimism. Whether we think about it or not, we are internally telling ourselves how we are doing from moment to moment, predicting how successfully things are going to turn out, even directing our thoughts and behavior. By becoming aware of pessimistic and negative self-talk we can transform it into optimistic positive internal communication. Several times during the day internally tell yourself positive, optimistic things ("things at work will go well").

We know it's hard to believe, but by practicing these self-talk exercises you can learn to become optimistic. As an example of the effectiveness of induced optimism, you have only to look at the work of Martin Seligman, a scientist at the University of Pennsylvania.

In an experiment, Seligman tried to modify the attitudes of a group of university students who scored high on measures of pessimism. He divided the students into two groups. The first attended a sixteen-hour workshop where the participants learned to internally dispute their own chronic negative thoughts—in essence, they learned to silently argue to themselves that things weren't as bad as they seemed. The other group didn't attend the workshop and received no instruction on how to modify their thinking from pessimistic to optimistic. Over the next year and a half, the workshop participants were only half as likely to suffer depression. Learned optimism yields definite health benefits.

Seligman has discovered that people who push themselves to be upbeat enjoy better physical and mental health. They are more resistant to infectious diseases and more successful at handling chronic diseases of middle age and older.

In one study of ninety-six men who had their first heart attack in 1980, fifteen of the most pessimistic people were dead within eight years. Among the most optimistic, the death toll was only five out of sixteen. Seligman believes optimists do better because they treat themselves like their own loving friend. "The person might learn to say, 'Things didn't go well today, but I learned a lot from the experience, and I'll do better tomorrow.' My other advice for overcoming pessimism is not to ruminate about bad events that happen to you, at least not immediately afterward. I recommend that you do something pleasurable that will distract you from your troubles."

If you want to become a centenarian, start today transforming yourself into an optimist. Don't tell others to cheer up; tell yourself.

CHAPTER 10

Try to modify personality traits known to be associated with early death and disability.

ONE REASON FOR THE POWER of a strategy using brain-body interaction is that it lets us go for the longevity goal on many fronts. The beauty is that, even as we know we can't do everything at once, a multifaceted attack on things that steal away years yields proven benefits. Those benefits keep increasing as we live our strategy from one year to the next.

Often we find that the things harming us have been part of our makeup for a very long time—so long that we have accepted them as part of our personalities, cruel but immutable. But, as with pessimism, we can rid ourselves of these characteristics.

Consider our attitudes to the people and situations we encounter every day. Three psychological factors put a person at particular risk for heart disease, cancer, or other causes for a shortened life span. Yet by being aware of them and working on them, we can change them.

- *Hostility.* People with hostile personalities tend to produce more adrenaline and cortisol, two stress hormones, which leads to an increased release of body fat into the bloodstream. This is harmless if release is followed by an opportunity to burn up the fat by some hostility-releasing physical exertion. But under the conditions of modern life, physical expressions of hostility, such as the violent actions and threatening gestures accompanying "road rage," are likely to land you in court. Besides, most hostile people experience their hostile emotions in situations where they can do little more than get upset, such as sitting in a traffic jam or standing in the middle of a supermarket line that doesn't seem to be moving. In such situations, hostile people can only fume and fret and make themselves sick. They also die sooner. People with hostile personalities have four to five times the death rate between ages twenty-five and fifty, compared with people who are less prone to habitual hostility.

- *Depression.* Depressed people often exhibit impaired immune functioning. Natural killer cells and cytotoxic T lymphocyte populations—key components of the body's infection defenses against cancer—are lowered in depression. That makes the depressed person more susceptible to developing cancer. It's both tasteless and cruel to tell a cancer patient to "cheer up," but it's a fact that treatment for depression, even if that treatment involves nothing more than group psychotherapy, prolongs life. Among woman suffering from breast cancer, for instance, those who participate in group psychotherapy live longer than those not involved in the treatment. A similar benefit is also observed in patients with malignant melanoma, a skin disease that often rapidly kills the patient. Among the melanoma patients, psychotherapy produces an increase in natural killer-cell activity. This increased survival is considered a result of changes in immunity. Both the breast cancer and melanoma results strongly suggest that reducing stress and improving mood may prolong the life of a person with cancer.

In regard to heart disease, depressed people are two to three times more likely to die of heart disease or outright heart attacks when they are followed over many years. And people who suffer a heart attack while depressed, or who become depressed in the aftermath of a heart attack, are much more likely to die in the next six months to two years than heart attack victims who are not depressed.

- *Social isolation.* We are inherently social animals, and sociability exerts a positive effect on hormone secretions and the patterning of the autonomic nervous system. People who have few social contacts and who report little pleasure in the company of others die prematurely. For instance, survival after heart attack and cancer is lessened in people with few friends. Even keeping a pet reduces the likelihood of death and disability: talking and tending to a dog or cat lowers pet owners' blood pressure and slows their pulse.

The good news is that personality traits are not set in stone. Sure, some of them are hard to change. But psychologists agree that we can modify any personality trait if we want to badly enough.

Depression, particularly later in life, is biochemically rather than psychologically caused. Antidepressant medications are effective in reversing the depression, often with the help of supportive psychotherapy focused on day-to-day living rather than explorations into the distant past.

While feelings of hostility and social isolation may also respond to drugs, most experts recommend additional psychotherapy aimed at changing thoughts and attitudes. Until comparatively recently, psychotherapy was long, arduous, expensive, and—worst of all—didn't always justify the time and resources expended. But cognitive therapy is the newly preferred approach, and it is very different. The emphasis in this shorter-term therapy is on modifying self-defeating and unhealthy attitudes by confronting and changing them in specific situations. For instance, even generally hostile people aren't hostile all the time, only in certain circumstances. Cognitive therapy aims at helping the hostile or isolated person to examine why he or she becomes hostile around others and doesn't enjoy socializing.

Cognitive therapy involves weekly sessions with a therapist. In therapy the person is taught to become aware of negative thoughts as they arise. For instance, a hostile person may be responding to what he perceives as the hostility of others. Silence or an absence of eye contact may be wrongly interpreted as evidence of unfriendliness. In cognitive therapy the person is taught to "reality-check" such perceptions before rushing to judgment. A simple query such as "Is everything all right?" may elicit the information that the other person is not being unfriendly but is merely mentally preoccupied.

Even though a change in personality may be difficult to achieve, cognitive therapy can change not only how a person interprets the people and events he or she encounters but also the emotions and behaviors that follow.

On many occasions inescapable negative experiences can be transformed. The enforced physical limitations accompanying a mild heart attack or ruptured lumbar disc can be seen as an opportunity to take stock of one's relationships with family and one's occupational plans for the future. The key point is to replace negative, self-limiting thoughts with more positive, empowering ones.

Cognitive therapy doesn't preach that every cloud has a silver lining. Some experiences are painful and difficult and must be accepted. Learning acceptance is one of the goals of cognitive therapy, a goal that seems to come easier to successfully aging people. But acceptance doesn't imply morbid resignation to an inexorable fate. One can always control one's attitude to whatever fate has in store.

Of course, many people have learned over their lifetime to successfully transform their thought patterns without the help of psychotherapy. The goal, with or without professional help, is to alter those thought patterns or habits of mind that worsen psychological, social, or physical disturbances.

Perhaps the commonest, and certainly one of the most destructive habits of mind, is just plain worry. There isn't a moment of the day when any of us can't find something to worry about. Yet in most instances, the worry accomplishes nothing other than undermining our peace of mind. Hillie Mahoney came up with a solution to this dilemma. "At a certain point in my life, I realized that the greater number of things I had worried about in the past had never come to pass. Conversely, when challenging things did come along, I often didn't handle them as well, nor was I as strong as I might have been had I not worried needlessly. Therefore, whenever I now catch myself worrying, I remind myself that it's a fruitless and debilitating emotion and the only things I can control are my feelings and thoughts and my responses."

And you know what? You can do that, too.

CHAPTER 11

Try to develop and express a healthy sense of humor.

IF YOU HAVE NEVER SEEN DAVID, you should know that he is tall and muscular, with a personal demeanor of vigor and drive that is a source of constant comment among friends and acquaintances. You will remember also, as he mentioned earlier, that he had heart surgery. But the audience he stood before a couple of years later saw only the exterior. He made his speech—on brain research and its gift of longevity—and a question-and-answer session followed. A young man asked, a bit skeptically: "Sir, what do you think you'll be looking forward to when you're eighty-five?" David didn't hesitate: "Eighty-six," he replied, to a ripple of surprised chuckles.

He's still pleased at how quick that one came out, but the story also has two lessons in it. One is that things that might disturb your internal tranquillity are very good candidates to be laughed away. The other is that a healthy expression of humor isn't made at somebody else's expense. Every politician knows that self-derogating wit is the most effective kind. Sure, humor can sometimes be wry and biting, but the healthiest humor causes other people to burst into laughter rather than wince or feel uncomfortable.

Unfortunately, some people use humor to hurt and wound. You can probably think of examples among your friends or even in your own family: the person who manages to get in a string of insults accompanied by a smile so thin it fails to conceal the underlying hostility. And if confronted about their hostile, hurtful "humor," such persons have a stock reply: "But I was only kidding. What's the matter, can't you take a joke? Lighten up." That kind of "humor" is actually hostile wit, doesn't benefit anybody, and serves as only a veiled means of expressing ill will.

Humor serves as an antidote for many things in contemporary life we can do little about. Our longtime friend Norman Cousins captured the dilemma in his 1979 book *Anatomy of an Illness:*

"The war against microbes has been largely won, but the struggle for equanimity is being lost. It is not just the congestion outside us—a congestion of people and ideas and issues—but our inner congestion that is hurting us. Our experiences come at us in such profusion and from so many different directions that they are never really sorted out, much less absorbed. The result is clutter and confusion. We gorge our senses and starve the sensitivities."

In his search for equanimity Cousins discovered the physical and mental benefits of humor and laughter. Each day while under treatment for a degenerative immune system disease, Cousins laughed his way through reruns of Allan Funt's *Candid Camera* and Marx Brothers and Three Stooges movies.

"I made the joyous discovery that ten minutes of genuine laughter had an anaesthetic effect and would give me at least two hours of pain-free sleep. When the painkilling effect of the laughter wore off, we would switch on the motion-picture projector again and, not infrequently, it would lead to another pain-free interval."

Today Cousins's observations can be explained scientifically.

Laughing at movies or videos leads to a measurable decrease in the stress hormone epinephrine. Dr. Lee Burk, a researcher at the Loma Linda School of Medicine in Loma Linda, California, finds that laughter boosts the immune system by increasing the body's level of T cells, a major player in the body's defenses against viruses and other infectious agents. A hearty laugh speeds up the heart rate, improves circulation, and works enough muscles to qualify for an aerobic exercise.

"We have laboratory evidence that mirthful laughter stimulates most of the major physiologic systems of the body," says psychiatrist William Fry, one of the country's leading experts on humor and health.

There is even some preliminary research suggesting that humor appreciation integrates and balances activity in both hemispheres of the brain. Humor is also infectious: Exposure to the laughter of other people makes you want to laugh along with them. Psychologists at Middlesex University in England studied the responses of people listening to a recording of a radio comedy. They compared one group listening to the program to the accompaniment of audience laughter and another group listening to the same show without the audience laughter. Those participants who listened with the background laughter present found the show funnier and more enjoyable. They also laughed and smiled more. Television producers have realized this for years: Sound tracks of audience laughter increase the likelihood of inducing laughter in the television viewer. "Canned" laughter works.

Psychologists at the University of Akron found a positive relationship between humor appreciation and longevity. As steps along the way to a longer, fuller life, psychiatrist Christian Hagaseth III suggests the following affirmations of positive humor that we should all try to practice:

1. I am determined to use my humor for positive, playful, uplifting, healing and loving purposes.

2. I will take myself lightly while I take my work seriously.

3. I will not seek to be offended by others' attempts at humor. When in doubt, I will see others as meaning well.

4. I refuse to use my humor to camouflage hostility or prejudice.

5. I will be eternally vigilant for the jokes and absurdities of the universe, and I will share my observations with my companions in life.

6. In the midst of adversity, I will continue to use my humor to cope, to survive, to heal, to grow, and to pass on loving kindness.

In Mumbai, India, thirty-seven laughing clubs exist. The members breathe deeply, reach for the sky to reduce their inhibitions, and force a "ho, ho, ha, ha" until all of the members are laughing uproariously. According to the club's founder, Dr. Madan Kataria, laughter is contagious, healthful, and reduces stress.

Even more importantly, humor increases your chances of becoming a centenarian.

CHAPTER 12

B*e proud of your brain. As you grow older, your brain performs better in the areas that are most important for success in the last third of your life.*

"I'M ALWAYS AFRAID I'm going to have a 'senior moment'!" Hillie Mahoney says with a laugh, about her rare experience of a momentary lapse of memory for someone's name. Although she jokes about it, the conventional wisdom about our mental performance after age fifty often leads to problems.

For years, companies and institutions operated on the mistaken notion that when it came to performance, younger meant better. Younger workers were considered more energetic, better able to work longer and harder hours, and more capable of learning new technologies faster. This line of thinking became so entrenched that in the early 1990s, employers began laying off older workers just because they were older. In some instances, "older" meant anybody older than forty-five.

In 1992 the Equal Employment Opportunity Commission received more than 20,000 age-discrimination complaints. With each succeeding year the number of complaints has fallen, thanks to more evenhanded enforcement of age discrimination complaints. Since 1993 the complaints have fallen 21 percent and are expected to drop another 35 percent by 2000 (assuming, of course, a strong economy).

As a result of age-discrimination monitoring, more people over age fifty-five are keeping their jobs. In July 1997, the jobless rate for the fifty-five-and-older set fell to a seven-year low, hitting 3 percent. Five years earlier the rate was 5.3 percent, according to the U.S. Bureau of Labor Statistics. Employers and workers alike are beginning to recognize the value of an older, healthier worker with a long track record of accomplishment. Again, the biggest winners are workers in their fifties. From July 1995 to July 1997, their numbers increased 12 percent, compared to a 3.8 percent rise during the same two-year span for all workers.

Another reason why legislation against age discrimination succeeded, we believe, is that it's based on sound principles about the human brain. The brain of a person forty-five years of age or older can outperform that of a younger counterpart when it comes to what really counts at the highest levels of performance.

For one thing, older workers are more experienced, and experience counts in making long-term management decisions. The medical and legal professions have recognized this for years: The more complicated your medical or legal problem, the more likely an older, experienced doctor or lawyer will be involved at some level.

Increasing age involves a trade-off in terms of brain functioning. It's true that the older brain often takes longer to process a given amount of information or to memorize, or even call to mind, an exact piece of information. Neuroscientists have confirmed all of this through testing of older persons and comparing their performance with that of younger people. So if you're over forty-five, don't be disappointed if you're outperformed in a game such as Trivial Pursuit by players a decade or more your junior.

However, if the challenge is a more encompassing one, demanding the balancing of several competing interests, then the older, more experienced worker has the edge. In recognition of this fact, by 1997, many companies had begun rehiring older employees laid off only a few years before. This benefits company and employee equally. After a few years of disillusionment about retirement, the former executive may be eager to get back to the challenges of the work atmosphere.

On occasion, the returning worker may be hired in a related area. For instance, a urologist known to Richard retired from his medical practice and took a position at a medical school teaching, not urology, but medical ethics and history—two interests he had nourished during his practice career.

Changes in the Brain

Whether working, retired, or reentering the workplace after a temporary "retirement," an older person can expect changes in certain aspects of brain functioning. Among the functional changes that occur in the healthy, mature brain are:

- Some mild decrease in what psychologists refer to as "fluid intelligence." This involves the gathering and use of new information. It may involve learning a new language, or accommodating to recent changes in the work environment. This slight drop-off in fluid intelligence with age is thought to result from the loss that we mentioned in chapter 7, of some cells in the areas of the brain beneath the cortex (the subcortical nuclei) that give us enthusiasm and general "get up and go" energy. With aging, this loss of cells also affects attention and concentration, making it harder to stick with a task and put everything else out of mind.

The good news is that slippage in fluid intelligence can be made up for by deliberate acts of the will: You can break learning sessions into shorter segments, and judiciously use caffeine-containing products such as coffee, tea, and some sodas. Crystallized intelligence (knowledge), in contrast, shows no change with aging. In fact, we know more as we age, thanks to the simple fact that we have lived longer and have seen more.

Another surprising piece of good news about learning and aging turned up in imaging studies done at the National Institutes of Health in 1997. Brain scans of older and younger healthy volunteers found that "motor learning"—learning new movements—is as fast and as complete in older people as in young people. So if you are in good shape, you can learn to tap-dance after all.

- Memory for proper names may be affected. This is perfectly normal and even has a fancy name attached to it: "age-associated memory impairment" (AAMI). A momentary difficulty coming up with a name is the most common example of AAMI. No other aspects of language, such as syntax (the placement of words in a sentence), comprehension, grammar, or vocabulary, are affected. In fact, vocabulary may increase with age in tandem with the increase in stored knowledge. This improvement will more likely happen if you make deliberate efforts to increase vocabulary via crossword puzzles, Scrabble, and other vocabulary-enhancing activities.

- Visuospatial skills—your brain's processing of certain visual information from the environment—may show alterations, such as some loss of depth perception, spatial localization, and the rapid identification of complex geometric shapes. These changes rarely imply serious consequences, and most people don't notice them until late aging, when, for some people, these changes may make driving difficult or unpleasant.

- Problem-solving skills improve with healthy aging, simply because the older person, based on his or her experience, is able to take the long view. Seers and humorists have written for centuries about the attitudes older and younger people hold toward each other's problem-solving abilities. What better example than this sign observed by Richard at a country fair: "Tired of being harassed by your stupid, demanding parents? Free yourself by moving out, getting your own job, and paying your own bills. And do it today, while you still know it all."

- Concentration and focus, related to attention, are vulnerable to distraction. With increasing age most of us become more easily distracted and find it harder to "stick to" a project or line of thought. One way of managing this perfectly normal phenomenon is to work for short periods punctuated by frequent breaks.

Overall, the mature brain doesn't function better or worse than a younger one; the mature brain simply functions *differently*.

CHAPTER 13

Nourish your brain through a lifetime of education.

EDUCATION TOPS THE LIST of factors that scientists have found to promote longevity and the retention of mental acuity into the ninth decade and beyond. And we're not restricting education to degrees attained or the number of years spent in school. Formal schooling is only one measure of education, and sometimes not a terribly accurate one. We all know people—even very bright and successful people—who have never read a serious book since they finished college or professional school several decades ago. To them, education was just another step on the ladder to financial success, something to be endured until they could go out on their own and start making money.

No. The kind of education we're talking about involves a lifetime of reading, discussions, and a general questing after connections.

David says: "Education must link that which is enduring and timeless in our culture with that which has been invented—and developed—in the past couple of generations. Our society needs to bequeath to a new generation not just facts but also the *power of intellect* that created our high-tech world. We must do that so all children grow up able to understand that world—to work in it, to guide it, to make the decisions it demands of them—and to meet their responsibilities to themselves and their neighbors."

The most important component of lifetime education is curiosity. At eighty, the novelist Robertson Davies—who wrote more than thirty books and had three successive, completely different careers (playwright, newspaper publisher, and university professor)—had this to say about curiosity in the mature years: "Curiosity is the great preservative and the supreme emollient." Rather than emphasizing any specific area, Davies enjoins us to show ". . . curiosity about *something*. Enthusiasm. Zest. That is what makes old age . . . a delight. One has seen so much and one is eager to see more."

Education carried out over a lifetime allows us to know a lot about many things. Further, the person aiming at continuing his or her education doesn't decide ahead of time what is worth learning about. The best way to continue the educational process over a lifetime is to start in your thirties or forties with intellectual hobbies. This may involve, for instance, a curiosity about the Civil War or other historical periods. Or the interest may involve science. In the eighteenth century, merchants and others maintained active interests in astronomy or biology. Although much rarer today, many amateurs continue to make valuable contributions to astronomy, as with the recent sighting and naming of the comet Hale-Bopp, which was first seen and brought to astronomers' attention by the amateur observers Alan Hale and Thomas Bopp.

Still another great educator is a book discussion club, where the group chooses a book that all read and meet to discuss what they thought about it. When Oprah Winfrey added a book club to her show, she not only gave a huge boost to book reading but also probably added to the longevity of those who discovered a new love of reading and discussing books.

But whatever the specific field of interest you may choose, education remains the best single preservative of brain function throughout the life span. This underscores another truth about curiosity and education: Interested people are *interesting* people. They always have something to share with others, whether it is a story, an observation, or an intriguing question. This is as true at twenty years of age as it is at ninety. This is why we encourage you to sharpen your sense of curiosity at whatever age you may now be.

While schools and the rigors of professional life may provide a major impetus for education during the first two thirds of life, what opportunities are available later? Under development are ambitious retirement communities based not on age but on brainpower.

An example already under construction is Arizona Senior Academy. The conception of Henry Koffler, now seventy-four, and formerly the president of the University of Arizona until his retirement in 1991, this academy is designed to attract scholars, scientists, artists, and others for whom curiosity and education remain driving forces in their lives. This think tank (only half facetiously referred to as "Einstein Acres") will be located in the desert southeast of Tucson. It will feature seminar and computer rooms, private office space, a faculty lounge, and performance studios.

Another intellectual community is the Chautauqua Institution, located on a lake about seventy-five miles southeast of Buffalo. Originally designed to provide intellectual and spiritual stimulation for Methodist schoolteachers during their summer vacations, Chautauqua has gone on to become an international intellectual and educational center. During the nine-week season held on its 750-acre grounds, participants attend lectures on subjects ranging from "The Mystery of Good and Evil" to the likelihood of finding intelligent life in outer space. The institution combines the best of a Victorian-like summer colony—complete with the grand Athenaeum Hotel, enclosed by grand porches overlooking the lake—with a technologically sophisticated intellectual retreat boasting one of the most advanced sound systems, along with a 5,629-pipe organ. Richard has lectured several times at Chautauqua and can personally attest to the educational riches available there for the intellectually curious older person.

Our prediction is that "Einstein Acres" and Chautauqua will turn out to represent a national trend toward alternative educational institutions that concentrate on toning the brain—"brain spas," if you will.

Writing workshops provide another outlet for creative expression. If you don't cherish ambitions to become a published writer, you may develop a deepened self-understanding by attending a journal workshop. Here the emphasis is on ways of achieving clarity and insight into one's thoughts and emotions by keeping a journal or diary. Whatever your choice, more than 1,000 writers' conferences on almost any conceivable literary genre are available and listed on the Internet by Shaw Guides, Inc. (www.shawguides.com). Most of the participants in these conferences are not full-time writers but doctors, lawyers, accountants, and other workers forging second careers for themselves.

"Middle-aged people come here," according to Robert Boyers, director of the New York State Summer Writers' Institute at Skidmore College in Saratoga Springs. In an interview in the *New York Times,* Boyers elaborated, "They entered the professions [after college] and felt unfulfilled. Now they have decided to go back to their original passion."

Younger people, too, attend writers' conferences to satisfy curiosity, stimulate their brains, and increase their career options in a tight job market. "In the past ten years an academic degree has no longer guaranteed that a person will get a job, so people think you might as well become a writer," according to Boyers.

Theater workshops are one of the best-kept secrets among adult pursuits. Playwrights and other working theater people often teach these workshops to keep their skills in peak condition and, in the case of playwrights, to try out new plays with the aid of the dedicated amateurs participating in the groups. Besides being mentally stimulating, the various assignments participants undertake give them the added benefit of working in a group of creative, like-minded people.

But whatever the individual motivation or outlet pursued (schools, workshops, conferences, or individual learning), you can confidently expect certain beneficial results: heightened curiosity, the formation of new neuronal networks, enhanced brain performance, and an increase in longevity.

CHAPTER 14

B ecause the likelihood of becoming a centenarian depends on how success-fully scientists can cure Alzheimer's disease, stroke, heart disease, and cancer, learn as much as you can about pre-venting these obstacles to longevity.

S O FAR WE HAVE DESCRIBED more than a dozen ways for you to use brain-body interaction to take conscious advantage of your brain's role in your health and longevity. We will describe more before you close this book, but we want to pause to give you a look at the future for some important enemies of longevity: Alzheimer's disease, stroke, heart disease, and cancer.

David has long kidded doctors in nonbrain specialties that the purpose of the body is to keep the brain alive. Now, the flood of findings involving brain-body interaction has brought the time of kidding to an end. In 1998 the Dana Foundation begins groundbreaking research with a group of distinguished scientists from some of the most prestigious institutions in the country—Harvard, Cornell, and Columbia—to discover the nature of the role the brain plays in causing and preventing stroke, heart disease, and cancer. As that work progresses, it will add weapon after weapon to your arsenal against illness and year after year to your longevity.

How can such exotic work in the ivory tower of academic science do this? The important thing to remember about brain-body interaction is that, while scientists will learn to describe it and develop ways for medicine and behavioral changes to intervene in it, the control of those mechanisms is uniquely individual—a product of your particular makeup and experiences in life. Thus, as never before, you will become able to act as a decisive participant in the stability and enhancement of your own health and mental happiness. Meanwhile, it is already evident that research is enabling us to be more active in our own behalf against the worst enemies of healthy aging.

Alzheimer's Disease

Alzheimer's disease is probably the most feared human disease of aging in American society, destroying the integrity of your personality, condemning you to what Zaven Khachaturian, director of the Ronald and Nancy Reagan Research Institute of the Alzheimer's Association in Chicago, refers to as "the plundered landscape of an eternal present."

At least 4 million people in the United States, and close to 11 million worldwide, suffer from Alzheimer's disease.

The loneliness of patients' families from a lack of public understanding has long been one of the worst features of Alzheimer's. That began to change when former president Reagan was diagnosed with it and allowed the diagnosis to be announced. As David wrote in a letter to the *Los Angeles Times*,

Reagan "served us once more" in putting a spotlight on what Nancy Reagan characterized as a "very long good-bye."

Despite frequent claims to the contrary, Alzheimer's is generally not an inherited disease: most cases develop after age sixty-five in people who come from families with no history of the illness.

The mistaken notion that Alzheimer's is inherited stems from the rare instances—2 to 7 percent of all cases—when the disease breaks out much earlier in life in a person belonging to a family with a history of one or more other sufferers from the illness. These doubly unfortunate people, who develop the disease three or four decades early, have an inherited genetic mutation in any one of three genes. In essence, if you're over forty, the likelihood of your coming down with Alzheimer's disease is not going to be settled by inquiring into the health of your near relatives and ancestors.

Nobody knows for sure when the symptoms of Alzheimer's disease were first noted. Khachaturian believes that King Lear's loss of memory and episodes of disorientation were suggested to Shakespeare by some personal observation of Alzheimer's disease. If so, Shakespeare anticipated by three centuries the first clinical description of the disorder by the early twentieth-century neuropsychiatrist Alois Alzheimer.

In 1901 Alzheimer assumed the care of a fifty-one-year-old woman, Auguste D. Over the next five years "Frau A. D." showed a striking deterioration marked by memory impairment, disorientation, paranoid delusions that her husband was trying to kill her, and hallucinations.

Upon her death, Alzheimer examined Frau A. D.'s brain. It was smaller than normal and bore the signs of severe shrinkage due to brain cell loss. When he cut the brain into thin sections, applied a silver stain to the sections, and put them under a microscope, he observed that the neurons were reduced to dense, intricately tangled, thick bundles of filaments. In addition to these "neurofibrillary tangles," Alzheimer observed microscopic formations, called "plaques," of sclerotic (hard) tissue scattered throughout the entire cortex.

Today neurofibrillary tangles and sclerotic plaques are recognized as the microscopic hallmarks of Alzheimer's disease—the most common cause of dementia. Dementia is an abnormal mental state marked by severe dysfunctions in memory, language, judgment, and abstract thinking that is severe enough to seriously interfere with work and social life.

Over the past two decades, starting in 1976, neuroscientists have moved beyond Alzheimer's anatomical description to home in on the biochemical basis for the disease. In 1976 neuroscientists discovered that the brains of Alzheimer patients contained decreased amounts of an enzyme necessary to make the neurotransmitter acetylcholine. This reduction was in excess of what could be accounted for by normal aging alone. What's more, the greater the reduction in the enzyme, the worse the dementia.

Like all neurotransmitters, acetylcholine carries information from nerve cell to nerve cell. It is particularly important in memory. Loss of acetylcholine-producing cells from the hippocampus results in an impairment in the formation of new memory—the hallmark symptom of Alzheimer's disease.

A second pivotal finding was the unraveling of the chemical structure of beta-amyloid, the sticky protein that clumps into the plaques first observed in the brain of Frau A. D. Additional research showed that beta-amyloid is part of a much larger protein—amyloid precursor protein (APP). Genes that code for APP are located on chromosome 21 and are altered in people with the rarer type of Alzheimer's, which develops in one's forties or fifties.

In late 1997 neuroscientists became excited about new genetic findings. These suggested the prospect of a predictive genetic test for the more common instances of Alzheimer's—cases that develop in people's seventh, eighth, or ninth decades. Two susceptibility genes were identified on chromosomes 19 and 12, and individuals with variants of one or both genes were found to have a greater than normal risk for developing Alzheimer's disease.

Genetic variants theoretically make it possible to make a rough estimate of how early in life Alzheimer's will develop. But is it ethically justified to make predictions about the likelihood of someone developing an incurable disease?

"I do not recommend genetic testing for Alzheimer's because physicians do not yet have the means to interpret the results of such tests," says Zaven Khachaturian. "Besides, testing positive for the genes would not guarantee that a person would get the disease."

A less controversial use of genetic testing involves new drug development. It's likely that future drugs will be prescribed based on a patient's genetic makeup along with his or her symptoms. But to do that, scientists must first get a better handle on what goes wrong in the brains of people afflicted with Alzheimer's disease.

Based on several important recent findings about the workings of genes involved in diseases that cause adult brain cells to degenerate, Dana Alliance neuroscientists are now confident that treatments for Alzheimer's as well as for several other, rarer, formerly untreatable brain diseases are just over the horizon. Among the treatments already available or under development are:

- Drugs aimed at increasing the levels of acetylcholine within the brain. A shortage of this chemical that transmits the chemical message in key parts of the brain is characteristic of Alzheimer's disease. Tacrine and Aricept work by slowing down the destruction of acetylcholine into its component parts. Another drug, metrifonate, which acts by a similar mechanism, is expected to be available soon.

- Calcium channel blockers, which act by maintaining stable levels of calcium within the nerve cells.
- Trophic factors to help brain cells grow and survive.
- Neuropeptides, small neurotransmitters to enhance memory and communication between neurons.
- Protease inhibitors, which may stop the production of beta-amyloid, the protein that builds up abnormally and forms plaques in the brains of Alzheimer patients.

Neurologists and other physicians treating Alzheimer's disease can now call on several treatments that seem to ease some symptoms and may slow the progress of the disease:

Vitamin E, an antioxidant, fights free radicals by oxidizing molecules that can damage brain cells. Selegiline (Eldepryl) acts like dopamine and shows benefits similar to vitamin E. Most surprising of all, ibuprofen, the chemical that most of us know as Advil, seems to lower the risk of Alzheimer's disease. It may do this by interfering with the inflammation that is believed to play a part in the formation of the distinctive beta-amyloid plaques of Alzheimer's. Finally, as described in more detail on page 192, estrogen replacement therapy lowers the risk of Alzheimer's in women by 54 percent. It is thought to work by boosting acetylcholine levels and enhancing antioxidant protection against free radicals in the brain.

With all the complexity of Alzheimer's, are we saying there is nothing you can do to ward it off? In a way we *are* saying that, because the cause has been stubbornly elusive, and if anyone tries to sell you an "absolute" preventive, you should say thanks, but no thanks, at least for now. However, several well-documented findings worth knowing about can contribute to your health and mental sharpness, and many researchers feel they point to protective influences against the disease. They are, in order of the importance scientists are attaching to them:

- estrogen and anti-inflammatories such as ibuprofen, as we've mentioned;
- physical exercise, which scientists have found improves memory, probably by enriching oxygen and nutrient supplies to the brain;
- education and lifelong mental exercise, which scientists think stimulate development of more brain cell connections to carry on when aging or disease begins to intrude;
- taking care to avoid head injury, which has been shown to increase risk for Alzheimer's disease;
- stress management, because of the damaging effect of stress on a key brain structure, the hippocampus, which is involved in memory and affected early in Alzheimer's;
- good nutrition, which includes plenty of anti-oxidant-rich foods;
- and most recently, and still to be more closely investigated, a positive effect on mental sharpness, even in people who have dementia, from the herb, gingko biloba, as reported in the *Journal of the American Medical Association* in October 1997.

Present and future research make it highly likely that Alzheimer's will be understood sufficiently within the next decade to enable researchers to come up with treatments and, perhaps, even a cure.

Stroke

Currently strokes account for almost 30 percent of all deaths. Among women, perhaps one of the least appreciated health facts is that stroke kills *twice* as many as breast cancer. Present and future treatment will be aimed at preventing the secondary degeneration and death of nerve cells surrounding the area of injury.

A stroke results from any interruption of the blood supply to the brain. Either a clot may close off a major artery supplying the brain, or a blood vessel may rupture, producing a brain hemorrhage. In either case, the result can be a devastating paralysis or loss of speech or other impairment.

The good news is that strokes often announce themselves by fleeting reversible symptoms that, when recognized, enable the doctor and the knowledgeable patient to take preventive measures. Secondly, doctors can now successfully treat stroke and, in many instances, restore the stroke victim to normal. Doctors now refer to strokes and threatened strokes as "brain attacks" and consider them just as treatable as heart attacks. In many instances the stroke can be treated by agents that either dissolve clots or lessen the bleeding accompanying hemorrhage.

Success using the new treatments depends on quick action; in most instances this means obtaining care within the first three to six hours of a stroke. That is why it is important to know the signs of stroke: weakness or paralysis on one side of the body; disturbance or loss of vision; confusion or disorientation; trouble speaking or understanding the speech of others; dizziness; and loss of balance or equilibrium. Strokes can and do occur at any age; in younger people they may be tied to conditions as varied as congenital high blood pressure, pregnancy, a history of drug abuse, obesity, or adverse effects of medication for other illnesses. So a wise longevity strategist takes note of stroke's symptoms and knows what they are.

Even in completed strokes, much can be done. Already neuroscientists know they can prevent much of this secondary damage in the brain of stroke victims by controlling the accumulation of the neurotransmitter glutamate. Under normal conditions glutamate is the most prevalent excitatory neurotransmitter in the brain. But when it is released from damaged cells after a stroke and pours into the surrounding area, it acts as a killer. Neighboring cells die, and the area of damage extends. New drugs will soon be available that will limit the extent of secondary nerve death and damage. Such improvements in the treatment of stroke promise to significantly enhance longevity.

As for prevention, what can you do? Since stroke is an accident in the blood vessels of the brain, the rules for heart and vascular health apply to preventing stroke.

Heart Disease

Heart disease (along with stroke) is a good example of how quickly some of our most fundamental ideas about diseases can change.

For years doctors believed that heart attacks result from a combination of high concentrations of fat and cholesterol in the blood coupled with elevated blood pressure. Together they produce fatty deposits along the lining of the blood vessel walls—a condition called atherosclerosis. In this model a heart attack or stroke results when a blood clot lodges in the narrowed blood vessel, cutting off the supply of oxygen to the heart (heart attack) or brain (stroke).

Many scientists now believe that the basic mechanism may involve inflammation brought about by overactive immune system cells within the blood vessel walls. According to this new view, many heart attacks and strokes result from bits of scar tissue that have broken away from the inflamed blood vessel wall and then become lodged in the heart or brain. Most important, an easy, commonly available blood test can be used for the marker of this risk, C-reactive protein, and serves as a general measure of inflammation and the likelihood of a future heart attack or stroke.

Among normal men (the tests so far have been carried out

only on men), those with the highest levels of C-reactive protein are three times as likely to have a heart attack and twice as likely to suffer a stroke. Aspirin can protect against this—just one 325-milligram aspirin daily is said to reduce the risk of heart attack by 50 percent. But aspirin doesn't do much for men with low levels of C-reactive protein—suggesting that aspirin's ability to prevent heart attacks and strokes in men with high C-reactive protein is because of its anti-inflammatory, rather than its anti-clotting, properties.

According to another new theory, heart disease may result from an initial irritation of the wall of coronary blood vessels caused by the amino acid homocysteine. Dr. Kilmer McCully, a pathologist at the VA Medical Center in Providence, Rhode Island, believes that homocysteines act like an abrasive, irritating blood vessel walls and setting them up for a cascade of harmful processes.

First, circulating immune cells gather at the irritation site created by homocysteine. Next, cells in the walls of the artery proliferate in a vain effort to heal the irritated area. Growth of this "plaque" of cells results in a narrowing and eventual clogging of the artery, effectively shutting off the blood supply. Eventually pieces of this brittle, unstable plaque break off and, like logs drifting into a narrow stream, block blood flow in the major arteries serving the heart: your classic heart attack. (Or the pieces of plaque may cause a stroke by blockade of blood vessels serving the brain.)

While McCully's homocysteine theory remains just that—a theory—it offers marvelously simple treatment and prevention opportunities. Vitamins B_6, B_{12}, and folic acid (i.e., folate) supplements enable the liver to transform homocysteine back into its original form, the natural and harmless amino acid methionine. All three of these B vitamins can be gotten from dietary sources (although folate is mostly found in grains, beans, and greens—dietary components not terribly popular in our culture).

Probably the best course to follow now is to take supplemental high-potency vitamin pills along with 400 mcg of folic acid daily. In addition, the future centenarian will want to keep LDL (bad) cholesterol to less than 130 mg/dL and HDL (good) cholesterol at 50 or more. This is best done by weight control, exercise, and a low intake of saturated fat, typically found in hydrogenated oils such as margarine, solid shortening, and prepackaged cookies, pies, and cakes. If total cholesterol levels reach 220 or higher, you probably will need medication in addition to dietary changes. Aggressive measures to keep blood pressure under control should be undertaken whatever the total cholesterol level.

New drugs are coming on the market that stop blood clots by preventing blood platelets from clumping together. With less clumping the blood is thinner and less likely to clog the coronary arteries, resulting in the infarction (death) of heart muscle. One platelet-thinning drug reduced heart attacks and deaths by 10 percent in patients coming to emergency rooms complaining of violent chest pains.

Cardiologists estimate that antiplatelet drugs have the potential to prevent 7,000 to 10,000 heart attacks and deaths per year. Within the next five years look for other, even more effective drugs that will either prevent heart attacks or decrease the damage in patients already in the throes of a heart attack.

In all, these promising findings suggest that we can now do quite a bit about heart disease, stroke, Alzheimer's disease, and other illnesses that cut deep swathes into the population of people eligible to become centenarians.

Cancer

But when on the subject of preventable deaths, we would be remiss not to speak about cancer, which kills more people annually than AIDS, accidents, and homicides *combined*. The greatest risk factor for developing cancer? Age. People aged sixty-five or older are ten times more likely than younger persons to develop cancer.

Since the cancer risk increases with age, and since the population as a whole is living longer, we can expect to see a rise in the incidence of cancer in the future. Fortunately, we now have knowledge that can reduce our chances of getting cancer and enable us to be diagnosed early enough for a cure.

According to a national panel of experts convened by the American Cancer Society, these are the steps to take to reduce your cancer risks:

- Increased consumption of fruits, vegetables, and whole grains
- Decreased consumption of high-fat foods, especially from animal sources
- Increased physical activity
- Limited alcohol consumption for those who drink
- No smoking
- Limited sun exposure
- Regular health exams combined with prompt attention to the established warning signs of cancer.

If these steps are taken, the chances of coming down with cancer can be lessened considerably.

Of course, we're not suggesting that you become your own doctor. But some familiarity with the illnesses mentioned in this chapter may help you to recognize health problems at an early stage. You'll also become a better, more knowledgeable patient who can communicate essential information to your doctor. Finally, knowledge of these illnesses helps in the recognition of risk factors and what you can do to help yourself and others to stay well.

So far we have concentrated on brain-body-life modifications. In the next part we tell you how to apply this knowledge daily.

PART THREE

Use Your Brain for Longevity

CHAPTER 15

Life is not a spectator sport; step out
of the stands and do something now to
increase your chances for a long life and
change our national attitudes toward
aging.

ONE VARIATION OF LIFE-AS-SPECTATOR-SPORT involves
nostalgia for the past. But when somebody talks about the
"good old days," we're curious about his or her frame of reference. In the 1930s we had the Great Depression; a major war in
the 1940s; Korea and the Cold War in the 1950s; Vietnam, cam-
pus turmoil, and a general distrust between generations in the
1960s; inflation and a spreading of Arab-Israeli tensions in the
1970s; and the savings-and-loan failures coupled with a burgeoning national debt in the 1980s. Now, in the 1990s, we have
the threat of increasing social disruption, moral bankruptcy,
and a general coarsening of life.
    So when were the "good old days"? The only sensible answer
is that the good old days are not in the past but evolving now.

The only good old days any of us are going to experience are happening right now.

David has a favorite dinner party question: Name the two most profound and powerful influences during the past twenty years on our daily lives today. The answers range from atomic power to television to the ending of the Cold War. Few people come up with the two factors that have affected the greatest number of people in our lifetime: first, the women's movement, and second, the lengthening of the human life span.

Women are now in the Congress; a woman is secretary of state of the United States; women are heading departments and chairing committees in our medical and law schools; women hold key positions in industry and finance. Women are also wielding increasing influence on our national political elections. The "gender gap" may well have turned the results of the past two presidential elections. Expect this influence to grow. Within the next decade we will likely see the election of a woman president or vice president. The success of the women's movement would not have been possible in the "good old days" when women were severely restricted in their career and life choices.

Granted that as women have filled up the workforce, a trend of family breakdown has paralleled that movement. But we don't think the case is made for women in the workplace being the *cause* of that breakdown—too many other, sadder influences are more likely to be the reasons. Among them we would cite a societywide decline in moral and spiritual values, unwillingness to take a stand for right and against wrong, and the lack of a coherent image of "family" that most of society can rally around as a reference point for personal and public actions. But maybe most responsible has been our general loss of sight of the fact that prosperity, an unparalleled standard of living, and ease of doing most everyday things is the overlay—not the essence— of modern life. The things that mattered 5,000 years ago—love, security, care of children, individual responsibility in a community, and so on—has never changed and never will change. If anything, the greater power today's women have over how we get and use material gain gives them the power to help rebuild respect for and the integrity of fundamental values in everyday life. In other words, the same act of will that produced women's success can make living the hundred-year-life the most successful social phenomenon in human history.

The second most powerful influence on our lives is the number of older persons who are living healthy, productive lives into their eighties, nineties, and beyond. What's more, we now have the information necessary to make a healthful longevity possible for most of us. All we have to do is remain alert to the opportunities for life extension made possible by modern science. We can go from daydreaming about living longer to taking active steps toward making that dream possible.

The psychologist Alfred Adler once said, "Life is what happens to you when you're making other plans." All of us have a tendency to fall into this mental trap. Instead of remaining alert to the opportunities and challenges of the moment, we make other plans, run scenarios in our imagination about how we think things should be or how we would like them to be. But the future centenarian gets outside his own head and works with the here and now. Borrowing from golf, the centenarian motto is "Play it as it lays."

We Americans also tend toward a nostalgic view of what are "the best years of a person's life." We march into our most potent years looking backward. According to a survey by Louis Harris, most people selected one's twenties and thirties. Yet, if that survey had been done at the turn of the century, most people would have picked their fifties, according to a poster current at the time depicting the life cycles arranged in the order of "the prime years of life."

Why would most people today pick their twenties and thirties? Because we countenance a culture obsessed with youth, a culture that has no place for endings but only beginnings and middles? If that's true, then our attitude toward aging, at least as expressed in our media, is one grand cultural contradiction.

While Americans over sixty comprise nearly 17 percent of the population, they make up fewer than 6 percent of all network prime time characters and 4 percent of the casts of daytime serials. As the authors George Gerbner and Larry Gross put it, although older persons are the fastest-growing age group in our society, they "seem to be vanishing instead of increasing, as in real life. . . . Visibly old people are almost invisible on television." That last point is particularly intriguing, since older people watch more television than the average viewer does.

These beliefs carry consequences. No less is at stake than an entire system of values. "It is the meaning that men attribute to their life," Simone de Beauvoir wrote in *The Coming Age*. "It is their entire system of values that defines the meaning and value of old age. The reverse applies: By the way in which a society behaves toward its old people it uncovers the naked and often carefully hidden truth about its real principles and aims."

Unending vitality, youthful looks, boundless energy, ruthless competition for personal advancement—such goals are becoming decreasingly relevant for more and more aging Americans. We can and must try to change our inordinate emphasis on youth.

Included in the necessary change is the development of fulfilling activities in addition to work, coupled with an emphasis on social environments that sustain good brain functioning. For instance, elderly people living in retirement homes show significantly lower social activities when compared to older people living with families. Institutionalized people exhibit impaired thinking and motor functioning. They are also more likely to be disabled.

These results have practical applications. Those of us in the twenty-to-fifty age group must rethink our ideas about how best to care for our older parents and relatives. Most nursing homes and other institutions, as they presently exist, aren't solutions at all. When the brain is starved, it atrophies for lack of stimulation; death of the whole person soon follows.

The message is clear: When it comes to maintaining physical and mental health throughout the life span, families are important. They can't be replaced by institutions. Think of it as compound investing in the areas of love and intimacy. This leads us directly to the next longevity principle: the family dimension.

CHAPTER 16

Invest in your family dimension.

IT'S HARD TO FIND ANYBODY TO DISAGREE: Family life ain't what it used to be. As life gets longer, young people are getting married later. Fine; that deliberation about a big choice should ultimately lower the divorce rate. But at the moment, despite later and presumably more informed marital choosing, the divorce rate is higher than at any time in our nation's history. In 1960, fewer than three marriages in ten ended in divorce; today five of ten couples split.

Part of the reason for our dismal marital success rate stems from the difficulties many people experience in dealing with frustration, especially when they don't get exactly what they want in every situation that arises within a marriage. A successful marriage demands negotiating skills—something that many members of the no-fault "me generation" have found themselves struggling to develop.

Another reason stems from our tendency to demand the same variety in our long-term commitments as we do in every aspect of our lives—work, residence, lifestyle, etc. This simply isn't practical when it comes to a long-term relationship. A demand for ceaseless novelty works against us when it comes to choosing and keeping a life partner. At some point you have to make a commitment, probably best during your second quarter. The smartest thing you can do in diversifying your life is to stop playing the field.

The wave of the future, in the Longevity Strategy, is to frame your life in traditional family settings. It always amazes us when we see people making calm, considered judgments in their professional lives and yet acting impulsively when it comes to the single most important decision they will ever make.

Remember what we said earlier about that frontal lobe executive function that peers into the future and computes better than any computer where your present action is likely to take you? If you act impulsively, choosing a marital partner you have little in common with and don't know enough about, divorce is likely to be in your future. And divorce, in addition to all the moralizing things we might say about it, is also a bad business decision.

Divorce is the equivalent of bankruptcy: everything that has been accumulated together by the partners has to be redistributed in ways that are less profitable for the partners than if the marriage had stayed together.

The no-fault, me-first era is over now. Looking out for number one will leave you as the only one in the last-quarter ending to your life. And if you're all by yourself with no family and nobody who cares, it won't matter all that much how much money you have accumulated. Burton Singer of the Office of Population Research of Princeton University put psychosocial surroundings and family support near the top of his list of factors contributing to enhanced longevity. Both of these can be planned for.

Do your market research in singlehood; choose for the long term; then commit to marriage; have kids; avoid divorce; and raise your likelihood of having grandchildren. Following this course, you can expect at least a couple of great-grandchildren to enjoy, to work with, and to help as you approach the century mark.

But obviously marriage isn't for everybody, and the same kinds of positive experiences can be found in other relationships marked by intimacy: caring relationships that help fulfill our needs for inclusion, cooperation, and affection.

Establish a family, nurture it, make it your highest priority. When all else falls apart, after all, the family is the one thing you can count on to be the maddening, reassuring, same-old, same-old. It sounds so simple, but if we can believe divorce statistics and data on how few people are having children, it sounds like many people aren't getting the message. Remember: the goal here is to be a player right up until the end. You can do this if you plan properly now to protect your wallet and your intellect. In that way you can be a family asset, not a liability, later; and your family, even with all the headaches, will enrich your life.

CHAPTER 17

Build in a backup plan; diversify your career from the very beginning.

STOP THINKING OF JOBS IN SERIES, one after another; instead, think of careers in parallel. That means planning your vocation along with your avocation, and keeping them as separate as possible.

If you want to go into business, plan an avocation like music or art; if you are inclined toward the law or the media, diversify into education or landscaping. If you want to be a poet, think about politics on the side, and study it seriously. Diversification is the only strategy that makes sense in today's rapidly changing society. You fail to diversify at your own peril.

During his 1996 commencement speech to the graduates at Rutgers University, David said: "In my case I had to learn diversification the hard way. As CEO of Norton Simon Inc. I had built the company over fifteen years into a $3 billion conglomerate. My total compensation was $1 million a year.

"It was an ebullient time, with all the trappings of the office—the corporate jets, the cars and drivers, the corner suites, plenty of secretaries and staff, and above all, power. Then, overnight, it was all gone. No longer was I chairman of the multibillion-dollar international conglomerate I had built when in 1983 Norton Simon Inc. was taken over by the Esmark Corporation in an unfriendly takeover. Although very well compensated, I found myself without a job and no sympathy from my friends. The support systems were gone, there were no more calendars filled with appointments, and no place to go in the morning. Did it bother me? You bet it did. It was the first time since I was nine years old that I wasn't actively involved in something, and I plunged into the deepest blue funk imaginable. It was the most difficult period of my life. At first I threw myself into golf with a vengeance, rising early every morning to meet Gardner Dickinson, the pro's pro.

"During this period I also found out who my real friends were, and gradually, together with Hillie's support, I was able to work my way out of that funk and pick up on a lifelong avocation and interest I had in health and medicine. That is when I founded and funded the David Mahoney Institute of Neurological Science at my alma mater, the University of Pennsylvania. Several years later, Hillie and I, together with Dean Daniel Tosteson, founded the Harvard Mahoney Neuroscience Institute, and I started applying what I had learned in marketing and finance to a field that needed an outsider with those credentials. And for the past ten years I've had more sheer satisfaction marshaling the force of public opinion behind brain research into the dreaded disease called Alzheimer's, into manic-depressive illness and memory and spinal cord injury than anything I ever did as the golden boy or a boardroom biggie."

As CEO of the Charles A. Dana Foundation, David galvanized nearly 175 of America's leading brain scientists, including 6 Nobel laureates, into the Dana Alliance for Brain Initiatives. As mentioned in the Introduction, the alliance was the outgrowth of a meeting in November 1992 at the Cold Spring Harbor Laboratory of 35 of the world's most eminent brain scientists. The meeting was hosted by Nobel laureate James Watson, often referred to as the foremost biologist of the twentieth century.

At that meeting many of the scientists wondered why the public seemed not to care about so many important advances in brain research. David responded in terms that may have sounded harsh but make sense: "The public doesn't buy research; it buys results or hope for results." Rather than simply bemoaning the loss of federal research dollars, he suggested that the scientists should go out and hawk what they were doing.

His goal at the meeting was to help these scientists gain some perspective on how public funding works. Why are we as a nation not increasing our investment in brain research? the scientists wondered. David suggested to them the reason: scientists and laymen interested in brain research are not getting across to the public and its representatives the scope and hope of brain research. Drawing from his experience as a marketer, he reminded them of a truism: when it comes to investment, the marketing manager exploits the size of the intended market and sells the hope of profits to come. And, he added, "Once Moses came down from the mountain with the Commandments, somebody still had to sell them."

Words such as "selling" and "marketing" have a way of turning off great researchers. They consider such terms beneath their dignity, believing that public recognition of their accomplishments should come as their just due. But scientists feel differently about competition. Indeed, some of us familiar with cutthroat competition on supermarket shelves and sharp elbows in boardrooms could take lessons from the fierceness of the competition in some of our most prestigious academic institutions. That creative, competitive drive in neuroscientists can be transformed into marketing terms. To gain public support, we have to market the worth of breakthroughs in brain science. Neuroscience has a great case, and that is where the Dana Alliance for Brain Initiatives came in.

At the Cold Spring Harbor meeting, Mahoney told the brain scientists to give him ten things they could accomplish in the next five years, and he would sell them to the public. Here are the ten research challenges those scientists came back with:

1. Identification of the genes that are defective in familial Alzheimer's and Huntington's disease.

2. Identification of the genes responsible for hereditary forms of manic-depression.

3. Development of new medications and therapeutic strategies to reduce nerve cell death and enhance recovery of function after strokes and other forms of brain injury.

4. Development of new drugs and other measures to alleviate the effects of multiple sclerosis, motor neuron disease (e.g., ALS, or Lou Gehrig's disease), Parkinson's disease, and epilepsy.

5. Identification of new treatments to promote nerve regeneration following spinal cord and peripheral injury.

6. Development of new and more effective treatments for manic-depressive illness, anxiety disorders, and forms of schizophrenia that at present resist treatment.

7. Discovery, testing, and application of agents that will block the action of cocaine and other addictive substances.

8. Development of new treatments for pain associated

with cancer, arthritis, migraine headaches, and other debilitating illnesses.

9. Identification of the genes that cause hereditary deafness and blindness.

10. Elucidation of the neuronal mechanisms involved in learning and memory.

After identifying the ten research challenges, each brain scientist had to sign his or her name to the list. Those signatures and that list are now framed and hung on the wall in David's office in New York; the formal-looking document with all of those names written at the bottom attest to what these neuroscientists believed to be doable by the year 2000.

While brain researchers have made significant advances toward delivering on all ten of their promises, several areas that worry Americans stand out.

"In the past five years, the evidence that all forms of addiction are brain disorders has been building," says neuroscientist W. Maxwell Cowan, co-vice chairman of the Dana Alliance and chief scientific officer of the Howard Hughes Medical Institute. Of equal importance, ". . . there is evidence that many of the long-term consequences of addiction can be eased or even reversed once the addiction stops."

When it comes to learning and memory, prospects are particularly bright. "How the brain works to make and store memories is close to being understood at the most fundamental cellular level," says Cowan. Over the past five years neuroscientists such as Columbia University's Eric Kandel have probed the memory process down to the molecular level. This is already spurring pharmaceutical companies toward the development of memory-enhancing drugs that will help not only people with memory disorders but also those with perfectly normal age-associated memory impairment (AAMI). "Most of the answers to how the brain makes and stores memory should be available within the next five years or so," predicts Cowan.

Additional future discoveries about the human brain can be guaranteed to head anybody's list of fantastic intellectual accomplishments over the past fifty years. At the Dana Foundation, support for brain research during the past seven years has helped bring about some of the most exciting advances. This has included, within two or three years, progress in the areas of learning and memory, emotions and stress, behavior, pain, mental illness, addiction, epilepsy, multiple sclerosis, stroke, brain tumors, aging, and Alzheimer's disease.

Here are two examples of recent Dana-supported research findings about the brain:

- The brains of boys with attention deficit/hyperactivity disorder show subtle abnormalities in three areas; these form a circuit that is thought to normally inhibit disruptive and inappropriate thoughts and behaviors.

- Some people prone to panic attacks may be suffering from a dysfunction in the vestibular system (or "balance" area) of the brain, resulting in dizziness and the triggering of the rapid heart rate and increased breathing rate characteristic of a panic attack.

Other research promises to further our knowledge of the brain and, what's equally important, help relieve the human suffering brought on by brain disease.

David says: "The Dana Alliance was established to introduce to the world a science that is already changing it. Brain science is a brand-new frontier that has the most profound implications for our health and well-being. And the alliance is, to use a basketball expression, in a 'full-court press' to educate the public and embody the commitment of the researchers to the service of human needs.

"Winston Churchill once said, 'All my life has been spent preparing to be prime minister.' I feel the same way. My second career, in furthering brain research, is so much more important, but if it weren't for the first one, I couldn't be doing the second. Success, or a resounding setback, in one career can lead to success of another kind, in the parallel career."

In essence, David is in early-career mode all over again—and successfully using the same techniques he perfected in business: organizing, pushing the right buttons, networking, being positive, and making the right presentation.

In Richard's case diversification has not been sequential. It has involved balancing two very different careers. Since completing his training as a neurologist and neuropsychiatrist he has combined a successful practice in these two closely related specialties with the writing of popular science books on the brain.

To each of these two very different careers Richard has devoted equal amounts of energy. And while on some occasions the two careers have come into conflict—such as when he has to forgo writing time to go to the hospital to attend to a sick patient—the energy and rhythms required are refreshingly different. The activity of rendering acute care contrasts with the less physically demanding, comparatively contemplative mindset required of an author.

Richard's career diversification is serving him well now within the context of many of the changes currently being made in the way medicine is practiced. He is a firm believer in the primacy of the physician-patient relationship; medical care does not involve the selling of a commodity but the establishment of an intimate and caring relationship that may last for years. He wants to be there for his patients when they need him.

Unfortunately, governmental intrusion into the private lives of its citizens is robbing many people of the opportunity to choose their own doctors, maintain the confidentiality of their health records, and generally make the major decisions about their physical and mental health.

In response to these changes, Richard has shifted his major emphasis from medicine to his second career, writing. Rather than helping people one at a time, Richard is now helping many people by teaching them about the brain. This has been a gradual rather than a sudden change:

Richard: "Since starting my first brain book, *Premeditated Man,* in 1975, I have alternated the emphasis between medicine and writing—sometimes not writing anything for months at a time and concentrating on helping my patients. At other times, such as when writing the television companion books for PBS, the majority of my time was devoted to working with producers and directors and trying to put in book form what they were doing with video images. My patients were wonderfully understanding and helped out by seeking their care at such times from other neurologists and neuropsychiatrists in the community. But they were also tremendously loyal. When my writing project was finished they returned and became my patients once again."

At all times his freedom to control his own life was enhanced because he diversified his career from the beginning. Obviously the choice a person makes about career diversification doesn't have to involve writing. It can be in any of the arts, or business, or combining careers, as with his brother, Christopher, who is an architect and a lawyer.

The most important thing is to diversify your interests and aim at helping people. As David puts it, "Anchor your behavior in your opportunity to help people. That way you'll be focused on doing the right thing, not just avoiding the wrong thing."

By diversifying his career in ways that bring pleasure and satisfaction while at the same time helping other people, Richard has maintained a successful practice and teaching career at George Washington University School of Medicine and Health Sciences while at the same time writing twelve popular books on the brain and human behavior. Along with David, he knows firsthand that a vocation and a serious avocation can not only coexist, but also can serve as a stimulus for the other.

The Importance of Avocations

Don't confuse an avocation with recreation. Watching basketball on television, or surfing the Internet for the latest interactive game can be a lively part of life, but it's not a creative avocation. And don't confuse a serious avocation with a hobby; do-it-yourselfing is fun, and so are clay modeling and gardening and fiddling with old cars. Hobbies are ways to relax and to make friends, and everybody should have some; but a real avocation is a subtext to a career, and a part of your working week to pursue with a certain dedication.

"One can join a group or work alone; the essential, it seems to me, is that the work be difficult, concentrated, and definite progress can be measured," according to writer Carolyn Heilbrun in *The Last Gift of Time*. "If the undertaking is not to become but another daily habit, easily donned and discarded, it requires strong effort and the evidence of growing proficiency. The purpose is, I believe, to maintain a carefully directed intensity."

Ms. Heilbrun nicely distinguishes the practice of an avocation from mere dilettantism. Why is it necessary to make this distinction? Not only because it gives balance to your second quarter, but also because it positions you for the time that will come, in your third or fourth quarter, to switch gears. And then switch them again—you'll have the time.

Here's the "self-management" program suggested by psychologist B. F. Skinner in his book *Enjoy Old Age:* "If you cannot find the kind of work you have done in the past, try something new. It need not be something that appeals to you at first sight. . . . Look for something you *can* do; the chances are, you will begin to enjoy it as soon as you do it well. If frustration or failure bothers you, start slowly. . . . You may be surprised at how easily you move on to longer hours and harder work."

Former New York mayor Edward Koch has taken Skinner's advice to heart. He's now serving as judge on the televised *The People's Court,* which was revived in the fall of 1997 after a phenomenally successful twelve-year run that ended in 1993. Koch's mayoral talents are less important here than humor—and Koch has plenty of that. "The people threw me out and now the people must be punished." In its earliest weeks the show became a highly popular syndicated daytime show.

How do you know what avocation might work for you—especially if you are one of those with many hobbies and talents? One good way is to start noticing what you do better than most things, that you hate to quit doing, and that pleases you to know that others seek you out to do it. Something that does that for you has all the earmarks of a budding avocation. In all probability that has the necessary ingredients for a deeply satisfying second career

Another spur toward career diversification is sure to come with the retirement of the baby boomers, starting in 2011 and continuing to 2029. With 76 million boomers competing for part-time consultant positions, the competition for post-retirement jobs may be fierce and the payment correspondingly low. Historically there is good reason to anticipate such a turn of events. The insurgence of boomers into the work sector in the 1970s sent wages plummeting by 8 percent after years of steady increases. The same thing could happen when the boomers start to retire. With too many people competing for a fixed number of part-time positions, a consultant at a major corporation may be in danger of pulling down a salary similar to somebody flipping burgers in a fast-food restaurant.

The only way to avoid becoming marginalized is to start thinking now of how you can diversify and personalize your marketable skills so you are comfortably competitive. For instance, Richard is trained in psychiatry and neurology. But there are surpluses of both psychiatrists and neurologists out there. So what did he do? He is now practicing neuropsychiatry, a hybrid discipline that blends the skills of both psychiatry and neurology in ways that would be impossible for a practitioner of either specialty alone. Ask yourself the same question Richard did: what is it about my training and background that can set me apart from the competition?

The same self-knowledge guided David: The world is full of senior executive consultants and ex-CEOs heading philanthropies. But thus far, you can count on a couple of fingers the number of them who have turned their business acumen and expertise up to full throttle to support those who push the envelope of science.

The point is to not be single-minded about careers. Be double-minded, or triple-minded; keep a pot or two on your back burners. Not only will this make you happier and a more interesting person to be around, but also this attitude, we are convinced, will enable you to live longer.

CHAPTER 18

Take advantage of your opportunity to wind up a millionaire.

THE AGE OF ENTITLEMENT is coming to an end. Only a generation ago people coming out of college had worries about such potential horrors as nuclear war. But the one thing they didn't have to worry about was getting a job and keeping it.

Looking back to the 1950s and 1960s, the U.S. economy was growing at a brisk pace. Of all the world's economies, ours was the largest and strongest, cranking out goods and services in an environment largely free of foreign competition. What's more, the youth of the past generation could look forward to an expansive social safety net. Big companies vied with each other in offering generous pensions. Medical bills were affordable. If things didn't turn out as rosy as planned, Social Security promised to come to the rescue and offered hope for financial stability in the later years.

Today, all that is changed. For starters, pension funds—a foundation for retirement saving—are much less available than they used to be. Fewer than half of America's youngest workers have traditional pensions today. Nor can can they totally rely on Social Security. Despite some recent quibbling about when and if Social Security could go bankrupt (it won't), here are some figures nobody can argue about:

In 1945 there were about forty-two workers available to support each retiree. In the next decade, the figure dropped to little more than eight. In just ten years more, by 1965, the figure was halved again, to four workers per retiree. Now it's down to three. That means three Americans are working to support one retiree. What's more, that support can only become spread thinner, since the life expectancy is rising. If you were sixty-five in 1990, you could expect to live another fifteen years if you were a man and nineteen if you were a woman. But however many years between retirement and death, your need for money doesn't end and rarely drops below three quarters of your preretirement salary. That means your financial security is going to depend pretty much on your savings.

But when it comes to savings, we Americans are flirting with calamity. Among people aged fifty-one to sixty-one, financial assets now average $12,500. When this is broken down into racial and ethnic groups the situation becomes even more desperate: $17,300 for whites, $400 for blacks, and $150 for Hispanics. These figures suggest that many people aren't saving because, despite the difficulty in saving, deep in their heart they believe the government is going to be there to bail them out of poverty during the fourth quarter of their lives. Nothing could be farther from the truth.

The baby boomers who count on Social Security and Medicare will be disappointed. Those in the postboomer generation cannot expect society's safety net to support them in anything more than subsistence; they have to start thinking about supplementing that with their own personal safety net.

According to a survey by Tahira K. Hira, a professor at Iowa State University, half of the college student population is worried about how they will make out financially even before graduating from college. According to the professor, 87 percent of people between ages twenty and thirty-nine admit to such worries—which is probably why a report in October 1997 found that this group is saving more than are people twenty years older. What's more, they express a sense of frustration at not knowing enough about money management so they can make sensible investment decisions *now.* Despite their lack of knowledge, many of them seem to experience little compunction about piling up mountains of debt.

Of debtors seeking professional help at the National Consumer Counseling Service, more than half are between eighteen and thirty-two years of age. This indebtedness is the result of the proliferation of credit cards (65% of college students have credit cards) and the increased number of students borrowing money from the government to finance their education. To many of the X-generation, money management is as mysterious and daunting as predicting this year's Kentucky Derby winner.

The Principles of Saving

Much of the mystery can be dispelled by the application of a few simple principles. To the centenarian, *credit-card living is out, leveraged saving is in.* According to one of the best summaries of the wisdom of financial planners that we've seen, by Albert Crenshaw, financial writer for the *Washington Post,* a successful beginning to financial success involves the setting of realistic goals, careful record-keeping, and self-discipline. He suggests getting started early in a savings and investment program. But to do that, you have to know what you have and how to make maximal use of those assets.

Crenshaw suggests as a first step keeping track of income

and expenses by category. This doesn't involve anything more complicated than breaking out income and expenses. You can do this quickly by sorting through a few months' worth of check stubs and credit card bills. This should give you a good estimate of your income minus expenses. If it doesn't, then you're probably spending a good bit of your income in cash. The best way of finding out how much you're spending is by carrying around a notebook for a few months and writing down each cash outlay, no matter how small. You'll probably find that this information will now enable you to see where your money is going. Several available software programs, such as Quicken, can do this easily.

Next comes the harder but more important step: looking for spending that can be eliminated. In some instances it will be credit card interest (at one time a legitimate tax deduction, but not anymore); other common areas include entertainment, dining out, and "impulse purchases" such as expensive cars, clothes, and furniture. In Hira's survey, 59 percent of the students said that they buy things they don't need and often "shop till they drop." The goal is to pare down expenses to create surplus money that can be invested. Debt reduction is the most important element in this program of financial security.

Once you've reduced your spending below your income level, you can begin saving. Set aside an emergency fund, perhaps in a money market account, that you can get to if you need immediate cash. Since a home purchase offers tax advantages that renting does not, you will want to buy a home as soon as that step is financially feasible. To expedite that, start a separate fund for your house purchase. You'll still have to borrow for the house, but the more money you can put down, the less you'll have to borrow, and the less your interest expense will be. And don't kid yourself about the value of the tax deduction: you'll spend a lot more on interest than you'll save in taxes.

Next, look into using the tools the government is giving you to save, to avoid taxes in IRA and 401(k) tax-deferred savings plans. About 40 percent of all corporations with 100 or more employees offer 401(k)s, which allow you to sock away as much as 6 percent of your pretax income in a wide variety of investments ranging from conservative money-market funds to riskier aggressive stock funds.

IRAs and 401(k)s put your pretax money to work for you. In some cases your employer will match at least part of your contribution. Examine the investment options available under the plan and pick a good, broad-based mutual stock fund if it's available. In any case, use your tax leverage to make your savings grow exponentially. In this savings race, the tortoise beats the hare; by taking full advantage of the plans out there now, and more sure to come in the next decade, you need not be a rocket scientist to become a millionaire—in real terms—by your fourth quarter.

The secret is to invest regularly, even a small amount, and automatically reinvest all dividends. If you invest $500 a month in an account growing at 8 percent annually, you'll have $475,000 in twenty-five years. An eighteen-year-old who invests $2,000 a year into stocks in an IRA for just six years and then stops (a total investment of $14,000) can become a millionaire by age sixty-five—*that's* the power of tax-deferred compounding over time. The odds are obviously markedly better if you don't ever stop until you hit that million-dollar mark.

Start Early

Your most powerful assistant in becoming a millionaire is time. The earlier you start saving, the greater amount you can accumulate. A decade can make a big difference. Consider two investors: one starts saving at thirty-five years old and invests $5,000 a year for ten years, accumulating a bare total of $50,000. The second starts ten years later, at forty-five, investing $7,500 a year for twenty years, for an invested total of $150,000. Assume both earn 8 percent on their money. Most people when asked about this scenario respond that the second investor should do better in the long run because he put in more money each year and did so for twice as long. They ignore the most important part of the equation: the first investor started ten years earlier. When both reach age sixty-five, the one who started at thirty-five will have $725,000. The later starter will have only $561,000, thanks to compound interest when combined with earlier saving.

How should you be investing your money? This is not intended as a guide to investment strategies or as a substitute for sound investment counseling. Nonetheless, we would like to make a point about what is probably the most maligned investment tool available: common stocks.

Suppose you had been unlucky enough to invest $1,000 in the stock market at the start of the worst thirty-year spell for stocks since 1925. That period ran from 1928 to 1958. Remember that the period included the Great Depression, World War II, and the Korean War. Despite these financial and social cataclysms, the blue-chip companies that make up the Standard & Poor's 500 stock index returned just under 8.5 *percent* a year. That means your original $1,000 would now be worth $11,478—far in excess of what you would have made if you had kept your money in the bank at a standard savings-account interest rate

Over the past seventy years the Standard & Poor's 500-stock index has returned an annualized 10.7 percent, while five-year government bonds have returned only 5.2 percent, and one-year Treasury bills (which earn about the same as money-market funds or bank certificates of deposit) have returned 3.7 percent. Keep in mind, too, that annual inflation over the same period has averaged 3.1 percent. That's why people who invested in the market and stayed invested earned 2 to 3 percent more on their money than investors who stuck to more traditional, more conservative ways of managing their money.

Most of us who have avoided the market as we grew older have done so because we don't like risk. During periods of fluctuation and adjustment, the market can provoke anxiety. Nevertheless, the outlook for stocks over the long term (fifteen years or longer) is so positive that *Kiplinger's Personal Finance Magazine* suggests that if you have fifteen or more years to work before retirement, you should invest up to 100 percent of the money you have set aside for retirement in stocks—and keep it invested there.

If you put that fifteen-year figure into the perspective we suggest in Chapter 23 about never totally retiring, then the case for stocks becomes particularly compelling. Many baby boomers have realized this and acted on it. Over the past several years the baby boomers have been the primary driving force behind the explosive growth of the stock market. Unfortunately, as mentioned earlier, a significant percentage of baby boomers are starting to become more complacent about saving and increasingly likely to spend the money they should be targeting for savings.

According to the 1996 Equitable Nest Egg Study, the numbers of boomers trying to save decreased steadily from 1994 through 1996: 82 percent in 1994, 77 percent in 1995, 74 percent in 1996. Furthermore, those who are saving are saving less—only $5,000 in the year 1996 compared to about $6,000 in 1994 and 1995.

"Despite the fact that most baby boomers are uncomfortable with their level of financial planning," concluded a focus group report prepared by the government's Administration on Aging in May 1996, "they seem reluctant to change, perhaps because they are not sure how to improve things or whether or not starting 'late' is a worthwhile endeavor at all. This uncertainty and feeling of helplessness only fosters inaction and denial."

Another reason for the baby boomers' lack of enthusiasm for saving, some experts suggest, is their unwillingness to strap themselves in for what they consider a roller-coaster ride: stock prices wildly fluctuating from day to day in an increasingly volatile market. Don't buy into this mind-set. As mentioned above, if you invest in broad indexes, you can ignore the fluctuations and invest over the long haul, regardless of the level or short-term direction of the market. If you have picked basically sound investments, they will grow over time no matter what might be happening at the moment. You work for your money; make your money work for you. Over the past five decades investors who have followed that advice have prospered.

You can also build up your net value by sensible spending habits. Future millionaires live well *below* their means, according to research by Thomas Stanley and William Danko, two marketing specialists who cowrote *The Millionaire Next Door*. This was a habit future millionaires started early and continued all of their lives. They started out as skinflints: with an average household net worth of $3.7 million, they lived in homes valued at about $320,000. About half of the subjects had lived in their present home for more than twenty years. Spending on other things followed a similar buy-less, keep-more pattern. Most never spent more than $400 on a suit or $29,000 on a car. We're not describing misers here; the millionaires didn't deprive themselves. Rather, they avoided conspicuous show-off consumerism that only serves to pump up the ego and drain money available for wise investing

"The secret is to put money somewhere where it will grow

without your having to pay taxes on it immediately," says Stanley. Millionaires spend the necessary time weekly to evaluate their investments. Stanley and Danko found this to average about eight and a half hours a month.

A firm belief in the power of the financial markets also characterizes this group. They are focused on the long term; they are buy-and-hold investors who consider the stock market as a productive place to keep their money. And they have learned the value of patience and selecting stocks for the long haul. Almost 40 percent of the millionaires interviewed by Stanley and Danko had made no trades in their stock portfolio during the previous year. The financial strategy frees more time for the things that really count—such as family and friends.

CHAPTER 19

U*plift yourself by doing some good for others. Dedicate yourself to making a contribution to society.*

THIS IS A GOAL THAT EVERYONE should strive after regardless of age. It is particularly important for those of us who are at middle age or beyond. We're convinced that many of the most harmful negative expressions and stereotypes directed against older people are based on the belief that older people are takers and not givers.

"Burgeoning elderly populations threaten to overwhelm government benefit programs" is a typical headline taken from a recent newsmagazine. Obviously if a particular segment of the population is envisioned by the other segments as "burgeoning," "threatening," and "overwhelming," ageism and hostility can be guaranteed. Unfortunately, many stories carried in the popular media feed into this stereotype of the older person ripping off the younger generation. We are told of seventy- and eighty-year-olds running marathons, swimming 70 laps, and, in one instance, "completing 250 sets of crunches, push-ups, and head knockers." Of course, such exercise, and plenty of it, is one of the important components of the longevity strategy. But why restrict our vision of older people as engaging in nothing more than self-centered activities?

With the gift of added time brought about by their prolonged life, older people have the privilege of donating hours of voluntary time in a variety of activities to benefit others in the community. Traditionally this took the form of grandparents gently getting between parents and children and thereby providing perspective and some respite for both. An old joke captures the mutual benefits the old and the young can provide each other: "Why do grandparents and grandchildren get along so well?" "Because they have a common enemy."

But volunteering time isn't confined to people who are grandparents. Volunteering can benefit organizations, community activities, and churches, whatever you feel deeply about. A large-scale national volunteer effort is already under way. In 1996, 3 former presidents and the current president, 30 governors, and more than 100 mayors gathered in Philadelphia at a three-day summit called by General Colin Powell to increase the level of volunteerism in America. And if statistics are to be believed, volunteerism is already a way of life for many of us.

More than half of all Americans claim they volunteered in 1996, one in four doing so regularly; nationwide there are about 93 million volunteers in America. According to figures gathered in 1995 by Independent Sector, a group that studies and represents nonprofit organizations, those 93 million Americans donate 20.3 billion hours of their time. In Florida, many schools, hospitals, and community projects have come to depend on people who volunteer their time.

Nor does the investment of time have to be along traditional lines of service. One friend of ours, a retired accountant, volunteers several hours a week in the business office of his local nonprofit hospital. Other people combine their volunteerism with interests in the arts by donating their time to local museums, theaters, and concert halls. And many employers have identified community efforts, such as literacy programs, in which they give employees paid time to help others during regular work hours.

Unfortunately, only about 8.4 percent of the 20.3 billion hours volunteers work is given in human services—helping out at soup kitchens, shelters, prisons, and halfway houses. These are the areas where volunteerism can really make a difference. And it's important to keep in mind that volunteerism isn't just for the retired or the economically secure.

There's no more fulfilling way of combating loneliness, boredom, or even mild depression than getting out of your house or apartment on a weekend and helping people "on the edge" who don't have the luxury of sitting around worrying that their careers aren't advancing fast enough to suit them.

"I think older people, blessed now with this gift of added life, also have to make a contribution to society," says Robert Butler, founder of the International Longevity Center and neuropsychiatrist at Mount Sinai Medical Center in New York. "And we know that they are already giving millions of dollars' worth of voluntary time in a variety of activities helping other people, children, and communities. So I think there is not only the fun part of a healthy extended aging but there's also a wonderful opportunity for older people to make a genuine contribution to our society."

Helping others provides a sense of continuity and meaning to our own lives. And "meaning" means more later in life.

"There is only one solution if old age is not to be an absurd parody of our former life, and that is to go on pursuing ends that give our existence a meaning—a devotion to individuals, to groups or to causes, social, political, and to intellectual or to creative work." wrote Simone de Beauvoir in *The Coming of Age*. "One's life has value so long as one attributes value to the life of others, by means of friendship, imagination, compassion."

We're not just talking about older or retired people here. Both of us know generous young men and women in their thirties and forties who regularly donate time in the service of others. They report that their weekends now seem less empty; time weighs less heavily on their hands. Because they have moved out of their own heads and started thinking of others, they are now more interesting people to be around. As a result, other people want them as friends, companions, and even mates.

And you never know where your volunteer path will lead you: One of the first steps in the long road to David's involvement in brain science began in the 1960s when, as a chief executive, he decided to help push his fellow corporate chieftains into what was then called "social responsibility" and, to set the example, he invested time at New York's Phoenix House, a drug treatment center that is today one of the largest and most successful programs in the country.

The important thing, whatever your age, is to remain involved and productive either in the service of others or in cultivating, again in the service of others, one's own private muse. In that way, even if the goal of living to be 100 isn't achieved, the effort involved in doing so will carry its own blessing.

Consider the poet Dante, who wanted to live to eighty-one, the "perfect age," as he dubbed it in his *Convivioi*. Dante never made it to eighty-one; he died at fifty-six—off by a quarter century. Yet his accomplishments by fifty-six, notably *The Divine Comedy*, place him second only to Shakespeare in the canon of Western literature. If we can judge from Dante, the desire to live a long life can serve, however long one lives, as a spur to achievement and contribution to the world at every point along the journey.

CHAPTER 20

Nurture enlightened self-interest.

CENTENARIANS ARE RAMS, NOT LAMBS. But enlightened self-interest is different from selfishness. The selfish person is perpetually engaged in a zero-sum game—me-against-them conflicts where one person's gain comes at the expense of another person's loss. Self-interest, in contrast, allows all of the players to win. Consider the typical type A personality. He or she is perpetually caught up in competitive, hostile interactions with other people. That same hostility is also internalized—the reason why type A personalities are at increased risk for heart attacks.

But if the type A person can effect an attitude change—get rid of bitterness, give other people a chance—then major benefits are going to ensue for him or her. Risks will be reduced for heart attacks, strokes, and stress-related illnesses. That's enlightened self-interest at work.

Ridding yourself of negativity benefits both you and the people around you. If you are carrying resentments and anger inside, then you are in a perpetual state of crisis. By getting rid of that anger, you not only improve your relations with other people but also improve your own mental and physical health at the same time. Religions all over the world and in all periods of history have recognized this for thousands of years. Love for our neighbor, along with patience with his or her foibles, is a great stress reducer. As we discussed in chapter 8, anything that reduces stress enhances health and prolongs longevity.

Personal integrity is also a component of enlightened self-interest. The most hard-driving executives know this to be true: While deception, misrepresentation, and duplicity can occasionally offer short-term benefits, they wind up hurting you in the end. Other people don't trust you. They don't like you. They don't want to be around you. But when you deal with other people in a straightforward manner—keeping your word, not making promises you can't keep—people come to trust you and bet on you. They know what they can expect from you. Best of all, you come off as the primary beneficiary of their trust. They want to do business with you or have you as a friend. By playing it straight with others, you best advance your own self-interest.

According to a survey of our nation's youth taken by the Horatio Alger Foundation, a decline in moral values is considered the third worst influence facing today's youth (drugs and peer pressure came in first and second, respectively). This decline has a corroding effect on attitudes. We live in an age without heroes: When asked to name a personal hero, the most frequent response among the students was "no one." Over the next several years we expect to see this change, as part of resurgence in the importance of personal integrity. It will be our nation's youth who will spearhead this drive as they mature into adulthood.

The Resolute Will

Self-interest, at any age, is also furthered by the formation of a stable and reliable character. While good judgment and an ethical sense are important elements of character, even more important is a resolute will. "Character is a completely fashioned will," wrote the philosopher John Stuart Mill. The psychologist William James made *will* the centerpiece of enlightened self-interest. "Seize the very first possible opportunity to act on every resolution you make," he urged, "and on every emotional prompting you may experience in the direction of the habits you aspire to gain."

When it comes to enlightened self-interest, the power of habit can be as important as personal integrity, character, and will. No less a personage than Charles Darwin realized this truth late in his life. With sorrow and regret, he wrote of the personal cost he had suffered by neglecting the humanistic interests he held in his youth. Here is perhaps the most powerful passage ever written on the interrelationship of habit and self-interest:

"Up to the age of thirty or beyond it, poetry of many kinds gave me great pleasure; and as a schoolboy I took intense delight in Shakespeare, especially in the historical plays. Pictures formerly gave me considerable, and music very great delight. But now for many years I cannot endure to read a line of poetry. I have tried lately to read Shakespeare, and found it so intolerably dull that it nauseated me. I have also almost lost my taste for pictures or music. My mind seems to have become a kind of machine for grinding general laws out of large collections of facts; but why should this have caused the atrophy of that part of the brain alone, on which the higher tastes depend, I cannot conceive. . . . If I had to live my life again, I would have made a rule to read some poetry and listen to some music at least once every week; for perhaps the parts of my brain now atrophied would thus have been alive through use."

Enlightened self-interest makes sense not only in terms of psychological satisfaction but also in terms of brain function. Too late in his own life, Darwin realized a fundamental truth:

If we don't establish healthy mental habits, some of our most precious mental abilities will disappear, our brain will wither away, and, in the end, we will end up hurting no one more than ourselves.

CHAPTER 21

P lay to win.
Spice up your life with risk.

SURE, YOU ARE GOING TO MAKE MISTAKES, and there will
be failures. The important thing is that you learn from the
inevitable mistakes and not waste time resenting having made
them. Always focus on the positive. As athletes say in the locker
room, "No negative vibes around here." Negative thoughts
about all of the bad things that may happen can make you sick.
But good thoughts about what you can accomplish can
empower you, even pull you out of depression. Note the lessons
of the past, but don't let them gnaw at you, because what's done
is done. Just keep moving.

Too many people concentrate on not losing rather than win-
ning. There is a subtle but important difference. If you play not
to lose, you're always in a reactive rather than a proactive
stance. You worry about keeping what you already have rather
than moving on and getting something better. But if you play to
win, then you're freed from the paralyzing thought of failure
and what other people are going to think about you if you fail.
The truth is that other people are too preoccupied with their
own lives to give more than a moment's consideration to your
fate. When you realize that, it doesn't make you cynical, but it
does free you from fears of failure.

Risk-taking in one's business and personal life fits in with the natural, unpredictable processes and rhythms that govern our lives. Of course we try to deny the uncertainty under which we live, but in our gut we know there are no guarantees that we will even wake up in the morning. As a doctor, Richard has observed firsthand over the years the sudden catastrophes that can wreak havoc on the best-laid plans. In the middle of a staff meeting Richard once observed a young doctor reach up to his head while his face took on a startled, uncomprehending expression. He looked at Richard and said something inaudible. Two seconds later he fell to the floor in a convulsion. Thirty minutes after that, he was dead from the brain hemorrhage that had so suddenly struck him down at the height of his career.

Cancer, heart attacks, strokes, incurable neurologic illness— any of us could come down with any of these illnesses at any time. If life is so inherently risky, why should we be afraid of risk-taking when it comes to our careers, our portfolios, our personal lives?

If David had been afraid to take risks, he would never have left a good ad agency position at age twenty-eight and taken his first step as an entrepreneur. He started his own agency. "I figured that if I could do it for them I could do it for myself. It would have been a lot easier to just stay put, but I relished the challenge. I enjoy working. Running things, not just the financial end, not this end or that end, but hands into the whole operation. Understanding it and running it. This entails risk. So if risk is inseparable from success, why not accept it? Better yet, why not learn to love it?"

"Risk," of course, varies from one person to another. It may involve quitting an unchallenging job to go into business for oneself, moving to another part of the country, a change in one's pattern of investing money, or simply taking on an assignment you think you can handle, even if you never attempted one like it before.

CHAPTER 22

Flex your brain. As we grow older, we have to define our new standards for success. Develop a flair for dealing with this change.

AS CHILDREN, TEENAGERS, and young and middle-aged adults, our successes can be measured by fairly objective criteria. We either advance or slip back within the corporate structure; our marriages either grow in depth and richness or they end in divorce or estrangement. There is little ambiguity during these years. But as we get older, the criteria for success become more subjective and less easily definable.

Psychologist K. S. Kitchener pointed out several years ago that the challenges early in life are like puzzles with definite solutions. Like a well-structured puzzle, our early lives involve situations and tasks that are clear-cut. What constitutes occupational and social achievement and, as with puzzles, solutions are almost guaranteed if you apply the relevant rules and techniques. Further, as with chess or a bridge game, you do not question the rules and techniques of the game.

Challenges in later life, in contrast, are more like dilemmas: less well structured and less likely to be resolved by one "best" solution. What is a productive retirement? What is the best way to counteract the effects of aging? Should one control the circumstances and conditions of one's death? If so, what measures of control should be taken? There are no correct answers here, no rules or techniques for these dilemmas that guarantee success.

Dilemmas also differ from puzzles in another important way: in a dilemma one rarely knows for certain when a solution has been achieved. Not everyone, for instance, agrees on how success should be defined in areas such as retirement, aging, and the proper responses to disability and death.

Few people adequately prepare themselves for the ambiguous, unstructured dilemmas they will encounter with advancing years. When you no longer have to go to the office, the division between work and play becomes that much harder to maintain. There is less emphasis on competition, rapid responses, and technical efficiency. Success stems from more private, internally derived sources. Boredom, meaninglessness, and depression must be countered with a shift from problem-solving to problem-finding.

Problem-finding involves thinking in a new way. The emphasis is on divergent thinking and the development of wisdom—the ability to adapt and flourish under the ill-structured dilemmas that prevail later in life. If you're in your thirties or forties now, start giving some thought to how you will manage the life shift from well-structured to ill-structured conditions.

One way is to diversify your career by developing an independent avocation that is less structured. A lawyer who takes acting lessons with the intention of someday shifting to a career in the theater; a doctor who writes fiction and plans in the future to spend more time writing than seeing patients; an accountant who is simultaneously learning how to manage a gift shop—these are examples of how well-structured and ill-structured activities can initially coexist and then undergo shifts in emphasis toward the ill-structured conditions that characterize the later years.

Robert Louis Stevenson, in an essay called "Crabbed Age and Youth," captured the challenge facing all of us as we proceed through life's various stages:

"All our attributes are modified or changed; and it will be a poor account of us if our views do not modify and change in a proportion. To hold the same views at forty as we held at twenty is to have been stupefied for a score of years. . . . It is as if a ship captain should sail to India from the Port of London; and having brought a chart of the Thames on deck at his first setting out, should obstinately use no other for the whole voyage."

CHAPTER 23

N*ever retire. To paraphrase Winston Churchill: Never, never, never retire. Change careers, do something entirely different, but never retire.*

R ETIREMENT, AS MOST OF US think about it, is an obsolete term. Most of us mistakenly think of retirement as we do graduations and weddings—just another milestone in our lives. One day we're working and—bingo!—the day after our official retirement, we're home enjoying a sleepy weekend that never ends. If that's the way you think about retirement, it's time for a "Heads up!"

The traditional concept of retirement was never anything more than a fantasy, one that few ever achieved and that many who did realize it lived to regret. Slowing down, relaxing, spending time engaged exclusively in recreational activities—if this is your idea of retirement, you'd better change it.

For one thing, few people can marshal the necessary financial resources to stop working at sixty-five and continue their usual lifestyle. Only about 4 percent of people sixty-five years of age or older can do that. It is estimated that nearly eight of ten Americans will come up 50 percent short of the annual income they will need to retire comfortably. That's because people usually underestimate the amount of money they will need.

According to Marshall Loeb, former managing editor of *Fortune* and *Money* magazines, most retirees need 70 to 80 percent of their preretirement income to maintain their standard of living. A single person making $75,000 and who retired in 1975 needs 75 percent of that salary. Where is it going to come from? If Social Security gives him $1,199 a month or $14,388 per year (the maximum amount), that means he needs outside income of almost $42,000 a year in 1998 dollars.

With the average life span approaching eighty for men and eighty-eight for women, if you retire in your late fifties, your retirement savings have to last twenty to thirty rather than just fifteen years. And if you're aiming at being a centenarian, those savings have to be large enough to hold you in good stead for another fifteen to twenty years beyond that. You don't have to be a financial planner or an accountant to figure out that we're talking a lot of money here.

In plain words, you are not going to be able to retire at the same age as your parents did, quit working entirely when you do retire, or count on the government or your boss for much of your support in your later years. The solution? *Is* there a solution?

Eject the word "retirement" from your vocabulary. Think less of recreation and more of "re-creation." Get rid of the outdated thinking that divides life into neat little compartments such as education, career preparation, work, and leisure. Instead, look for ways to incorporate some of your re-creation plans into your present life, whatever your age.

As Ginita Hall and Victoria Collins put it in their book *Your Next Fifty Years*, "Instead of a single date in time or an age marking the change in what you do with your daily life, you must learn to think of lifelong learning, lifelong working, and lifelong experience."

Re-creation started the very first day you reported to your first job. Sounds strange? Think of it this way: Nobody works twenty-four hours a day, seven days a week—you have time off from work, right? What do you do with yourself when you are not working? What activities do you find interesting, rewarding, and exciting? If you have to think for more than a second or two to answer those questions, then the last thing in the world you should do is retire, whatever your income. You will be at risk of experiencing a frustrating, unhappy re-creation.

If you haven't developed authentic interests and enthusiasms in your thirties and forties, it's unlikely you will be able to do so after age sixty-five (or whatever the "official" re-creation age eventually becomes). That's because your re-creation has *already started*—what you will be doing after you've stopped going to the office will be only an extension of what you're doing now when you're not at work. In some ways this is a frightening prospect. But it doesn't have to be. Not if you start thinking of re-creation as a gradual transition, something like the transition from one color to another along a spectrum.

"Old age is like everything else. To make a success of it, you've got to start young," Fred Astaire once said. If he had substituted "retirement" for "old age," he would have been equally on target. It's vital that you develop interests and enthusiasms— things you care passionately about—*now* so that re-creation can be experienced as it should be: not an abrupt discontinuation, but the natural maturing of a process that started years earlier.

If you're a man, you have to take even more care in designing your re-creation. Thanks to centuries-long cultural conditioning, men look to their work for their sense of identity and worth.

Take Lee Iacocca: most of us remember him as the man who rescued Chrysler from financial ruin. Iacocca knows only too well the emotional cost of overidentifying with one's work role. When Tom Brokaw on *NBC Nightly News* interviewed Iacocca, Brokaw asked, "You had a lot of friends who were captains of industry like you. Did you ever talk about what to do when you left these paneled offices?"

"Never," Iacocca admitted. "And that was a big mistake. People are saying to me, 'I want to retire at forty or fifty.' I tell them, don't do it. Take it from me, don't do it. Your mind starts to atrophy if you don't stay involved. Life involves work. Retirement, it's for the birds."

After unhappy years in retirement, Iacocca learned something you already know at this point in the book: your brain works best under continued challenge. Endless rounds of golf or tennis or other recreational activities are not going to keep your brain in shape, no matter how much money you retire with.

"Money does not bring you the happiness you thought it would," according to Iacocca, who favors an automotive metaphor for what can happen if you suddenly call it quits. "You are going at full tilt and you are in overdrive and you slam your car into low gear. You are going to go through the windshield if you are not ready for it." At seventy-two, Iacocca formed a company to design and market what he calls the transportation of the future: electric cars, bikes, and scooters. He now knows from personal experience the perils of suddenly shutting everything down. "I should have thought it out better than I did."

Work and occupation are important to women as well. But so far culture hasn't conditioned women to think of themselves solely in terms of the office. Women—again generalizing—tend to be more sociable, more likely to maintain their contacts with friends, even former coworkers. As a result, women are less likely than men to complain of having "nothing to do" when one career ends.

"One of the 'constant factors' in men," according to Carolyn G. Heilbrun, is "a total inability to change any part of themselves but their appearance, even if they proclaim a desire to change. Women, on the other hand, are always undergoing change, sculpting their personalities and characters as if these were so much clay."

While Ms. Heilbrun admits to some irony here, it's hard to disagree with her point: men, on the whole, do find it harder to change, and they suffer disproportionately. But whatever your gender, all the extra time in the world will be of no benefit to you if you haven't done the necessary spadework to guarantee yourself an opportunity to keep exercising all the talents and skills you have developed over your work career.

Even more important, our brain has great difficulty adjusting to a sudden transition from a full, perhaps overly full work schedule, to the prospect of limitless leisure. The poet Charles Lamb, in "The Superannuated Man," provides a starkly poignant self-description by a man who suddenly finds himself with more leisure time than he had ever imagined. "I am no longer clerk to the Firm of etc. I am Retired Leisure. I am to be met with in trim gardens. I am already come to be known by my vacant face and careless gesture, perambulating at no fixed pace, nor with any settled purpose. I walk about; not to and from."

No doubt Lamb's superannuated man would have been aided by a supportive social network, good health, and adequate finances.

While planning a second or third career is important for people of all ages, it is vital for the baby boomers, the 76 million people born between 1946 and 1964 who now represent one-third of the U.S. population. Since one third of all baby boomers are expected to reach at least age eighty-five—a conservative estimate, we think—they should be actively involved in thinking about what they will do in the last quarter of their lives.

In January 1996, the first of the baby boomers turned fifty. Every seven and one-half minutes, a boomer celebrates his or her fiftieth birthday. By the year 2030, all of the baby boomers will be past age sixty-five. At that point, will they retire? Some will, and their mental activity will decline. Most will not, we believe, because brain scientists will make the case that mental activity is central to keeping the brain alive and alert. And the boomers will get the message.

CHAPTER **24**

B*ecome computer-literate and learn to use e-mail lest you lose touch.*

W E MEAN THIS SPECIFICALLY, but this tactic is also a metaphor. It means that you should keep up with technology. Nothing is more depressing and disempowering than to feel that the world is passing you by. If you are currently middle-aged and parked beside the information highway instead of being on it, turn onto the ramp. You don't want to be like the guy David tells about who was confronted by a friend. "What's with you? I e-mailed you eight times last month and you never replied." "Oh," answers the abashed miscreant, "my son was at camp."

You can enter cyberspace no matter how old you are. About 7.6 million Internet users in North America are age fifty or older. While this may sound impressive, only 1 percent of Internet users and only 4 percent of total online subscribers are sixty-five or older. What can be done to get more older users online? The American Association of Retired Persons has a web site with more than 1,000 pages. For the future centenarian, the explosive development of PCs and the Internet provides the means to prolong a useful and productive career almost indefinitely.

Sister Helen, a ninety-year-old Swiss nun, can personally

attest to the liberating power of learning to use computers late in life. After her recent retirement, she took computer classes. "They say you are only as old as you feel. That's the way I see it. The fact that I'm ninety years old now doesn't really impress me. I felt, yes, why not? With perseverance, I would be able to come to terms with this device and even make friends with it."

Sister Helen did come to terms with the computer and went on to complete her course and received her diploma; she is perhaps the oldest computer course graduate in Switzerland. She is now employing her computer talents in writing letters and design for leaflets at her local parish. Soon there will be many older people like Sister Helen who will benefit from learning computer skills.

Duke University Medical Center did a study titled "The Impact of Internet and E-mail Access on the Quality of Life of Older Adults." Older people with online opportunities experience enhanced social well-being and reduced loneliness and depression. The investigators suggest that "Internet training and access represent a promising intervention for preventing the psychological deterioration often associated with physical disability, and perhaps improving quality of life for older adults."

Here is one of the benefits cited by the Hudson Institute's *Workforce 2020: Work and Workers in the 21st Century:* "Because physical presence in a particular location at a particular time will become increasingly irrelevant, structural barriers to the employment of older Americans will continue to fall away." Thanks to computer networks, workers can take advantage of flexible hours and the option of working from home.

"Americans of all backgrounds will be increasingly able to determine their own working environments and hours," says the Hudson report. "The most successful firms of the early twenty-first century will find ways to benefit from the experience and talents of older workers." Personal business ventures also can benefit. If you get on the Net, you can call up the relevant information to manage your stock portfolio and discover new sources of supply.

PCs also have exerted a tremendous influence on private life. "E-mail is the perfect way to encounter the world outside one's own private domain," writes Carolyn Heilbrun, "without filling out any forms, enrolling, traveling, or revealing anything whatsoever about oneself unless choosing to do so."

E-mail is instant communication. If you're thinking about your mother or daughter, just sit down at the computer and quickly fire off an electronic note that expresses your thoughtfulness. E-mail makes possible a "catching up" with people who for one reason or another may not be available for face-to-face communication. Grandparents and grandchildren can keep in touch via e-mail instead of via letters, which nobody seems to find time to write anymore.

At a commencement address Richard attended recently, a college president expressed appreciation for the e-mail support given the graduating seniors by their parents and grandparents over the preceding four years: "Without those e-mails, some of you might not have put in the effort required to successfully complete your studies."

While e-mail can do a lot to enhance communication and lessen the sense of isolation, there are some hazards. Hermitism is one. Don't let anybody tell you electronic means of communication can improve on face-to-face personal contact. Psychiatrists are increasingly encountering individuals for whom the Internet serves as a substitute for the rough-and-tumble of face-to-face interaction with others.

On e-mail you don't have to dress up or shave or make eye contact with your correspondent. While that may be good in some ways (such as breaking down the artificial barriers that often limit communication—class, race, personal appearance, etc.), it also can lead to a blunting of our sensibilities. On e-mail it's all too easy to take on a general tone of easy camaraderie that may not always be appropriate. After all, we don't engage in the same conversational banter with the next-door neighbor that we do with someone we have known since childhood. Electronic communication is intended as a means of furthering person-to-person contact—not as a substitute for it. What's needed is the resolution and wisdom to avoid becoming either dependent on or addicted to this new vehicle for social interaction.

The writing of this book is an example of the marvels of e-mail and fax. Ideas and writings were exchanged between Richard in Washington and David in his commute from New York to Palm Beach to Geneva, Switzerland. Via fax and e-mail, each of the coauthors was able to establish communication with the other at any time. Thanks to this technology, similar collaborative efforts will soon become the norm.

But it is perhaps David's wife, Hillie, who makes the point most pertinent to the Longevity Strategy about this new technology. Hillie believes that our most important challenge is to conserve and wisely use the store of physical and mental energy that is unique to all of us. "Not everyone has the same store of energy; some of us are more energetic than others. But whatever the energy level, the important thing is not to waste our energy. We have to take control of our lives so we're not worn out by an energy-depleting lifestyle."

Technology both contributes to and helps resolve this threat to our energy stores. For instance, while phone calls can inundate us with obligations, the judicious use of fax machines and e-mail can come to our rescue. "I love the fax, because sometimes I'm a bit overwhelmed and don't have the time to take or make a phone call," says Hillie. "I'll send a fax with the essentials and promise to talk later."

Then there's the story of the modern, possessive mother instilling guilt in her offspring: "You never write, you never call, you never fax. . . ."

CHAPTER 25

D*on't turn to the obituary page first. Loss is part of life. As we age, our friends and relatives may die or become disabled, but depression is not a natural response to such losses.*

MANY OF US THINK IT'S NORMAL to become depressed as one ages. It's not. Depression at any age is a disease requiring and responding to treatment. But the incidence of depression increases with age, particularly among those no longer living on their own.

Although fewer than 3 percent of older people living in the community suffer from depression, the numbers escalate among people living in institutions: a 15 to 25 percent prevalence of depression is found among nursing home residents and a 13 percent incidence among residents of long-term-care facilities. What's worse, depression is often not recognized or treated because even many doctors hold the mistaken belief that late-life depression is normal.

The good news is that depression is an eminently treatable disease that should carry no stigma.

As we said earlier, David was able to pull himself out of a depression he suffered in 1983 and 1984 with the help of loving friends and family—and by having an avocation. By helping others, he was helping himself.

Not every depressed person can achieve recovery without expert help and medication. At some point the depression affects the brain's neurotransmitters.

Neurotransmitters are chemical messengers that are released from the axon, an extension of the neuron. They then travel across a tiny open space or junction, the synapse, where each neurotransmitter locks onto a specialized receptor. This linkage of neurotransmitter to its receptor is often compared to that of a lock and a key; alter either the lock or the key ever so slightly, and the lock will not open.

Serious depressions, depressions you can't just shake yourself out of, can be thought of in terms of neurotransmitter and receptor imbalances. A host of antidepressant medications work by bringing one or more of these neurotransmitters back into balance. How do they do this?

Antidepressant drugs work by increasing the amount of neurotransmitter within the synapse, the tiny space separating one neuron from another. For reasons nobody understands completely, depression lifts with this increased availability of neurotransmitter within the synapse.

The latest generation of antidepressants are thought to work by inhibiting a process called "reuptake." Reuptake from the synapse involves sweeping the neurotransmitter molecules out of the synapse and back into the neuron that originally released them. When this happens, less neurotransmitter is available in the synapse, and depression results in those vulnerable to the disorder. But the brain cell's reuptake pump can be blocked by an

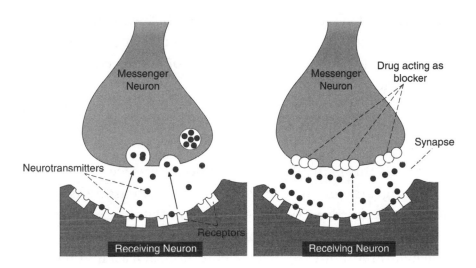

How antidepressants work: Normal reuptake inactivates a mood-regulating neuro-transmitter (left); an antidepressant drug blocks reuptake (right). From *Drugs and the Brain* by Snyder © 1986 by Scientific American Books. Altered with permission of W. H. Freeman and Company by Leigh Coriale Design and Illustration with permission.

inhibiting drug. Prozac is the most famous; it binds to the transporter for the neurotransmitter serotonin and hence is called a serotonin reuptake inhibitor or SRI. Other antidepressants block the reuptake of other neurotransmitters, such as dopamine or norepinephrine. In each instance one or more of the neurotransmitters stays for a longer period of time in the synapse.

Relief from depression can come when neurotransmitter action is curtailed in another way. This involves blocking the action of special enzymes that break neurotransmitters down into small chemicals. The most powerful of these enzymes, monoamine oxidase, converts the neurotransmitter into an inactive chemical that no longer exerts an effect on the brain. Monoamine oxidase inhibitors block the action of the enzyme and conserve the neurotransmitter. Thus more neurotransmitter remains available to act in the synapse and thereby exerts an antidepressant effect.

With aging, people notice a certain tendency to get blue

more easily. Everyone knows a senior who seems to have lost enthusiasm for life. Particularly among the elderly, this is an urgent problem—and a major subject of doctor education by the American Medical Association—because elderly people suffering from depression are the last-treated group. And yet they could be not only happier, but also a whole lot healthier, if their depression were treated.

Why is this particular to aging? Because as we pass beyond middle age, the number of cells producing neurotransmitters drops by as much as 60 percent. This translates into a dramatic reduction in the production of the neurotransmitter. Less available neurotransmitter results in depression, at least in some people. But this depression can be reversed by the timely use of an antidepressant that resets the neurotransmitter imbalance. In fact, serious depressions—depressions you can't just shake yourself out of—are best thought of in terms of neurotransmitter imbalances. A host of antidepressant medications work by bringing these neurotransmitters back into balance.

Many older people with physical complaints actually are suffering from depression. What's worse, the depression isn't recognized by their friends or relatives, and often not even by their doctors. That's because the older depressed person doesn't act or talk about sadness. He or she describes loss of appetite, lack of energy, and decreased enthusiasm for doing anything or seeing anybody. The older depressive is more likely to be reclusive and cantankerous. Instead of recognizing these personality changes for what they are—depression, not crabbiness—many people simply attribute it to normal changes with aging. Such mistaken "explanations" are particularly common if the older person has recently suffered a loss.

Certainly bereavement involves symptoms similar to depression. But normal bereavement is not accompanied by depression.

Depression and grief follow two different courses, according to psychiatric researchers. Treatment with antidepressants can cure the depression without interfering with the necessary process of grieving. This is important to know, since many doctors, quite correctly, feel that bereavement is part of the life process and should not be interfered with by mood-altering medications: there are times when it is appropriate to be sad. But normal bereavement does not go on for months and does not lead to reclusiveness and the depressive features we just mentioned.

Loss and its associated loneliness may be a normal part of aging, but depression is not. When it occurs later in life, depression is intimately linked with changes in the brain's neurotransmitters. Most importantly, depression responds to low doses of antidepressants. Failure to recognize depression in oneself or in others can lead to needless tragedy—older people have a higher suicide rate than any other age group. More than 90 percent of the people who commit suicide suffer from depression, either alone or associated with alcoholism.

An important part of the Longevity Strategy involves learning about depression, promptly recognizing its earliest signs, and immediately seeking help from a psychiatrist or neuropsychiatrist knowledgeable about antidepressants. Depression is a disease. Don't learn to live with it. Get help and cure it.

PART FOUR

Do Right by Your Body

Set priorities and stick to them, especially in regard to maintaining physical fitness. In the long run, it's the best, most efficient strategy for a potential centenarian.

SOPHIE TUCKER SAID, "The key to longevity? Keep breathing." But she was just joking—we think.

Work the longevity strategy by taking care of the body. Your brain runs your body, as we've shown you, but for a real shot at longevity, you've got to make the brain-body connection consciously and make *all* the breakthrough findings—including the purely physical ones—work for you.

We asked Donna de Varona—twice Olympic Gold Medalist in swimming, honored in the Olympic Hall of Fame, and a friend for many years—how serious adults could achieve total fitness. She says: "A good fitness program must involve mind, body, and spirit. Most of all, you have to love what you're doing. The easiest way to achieve that is to get started early in life doing those sports and exercises that appeal to you. For me, swimming is the perfect exercise because it combines stretching, endurance, and meditation. Usually I try to swim a mile or so three or four times a week. Of course, shorter distances would be sufficient for most people. The important thing is to find a distance that is comfortable for you and swim it regularly.

"Swimming must be combined with some form of weight-bearing exercise. Walking or light jogging are fine and can even be combined with swimming via some water jogging.

"The other components of optimum fitness are: knowledge about good nutrition and the application of that knowledge to your diet; regular stretching exercises such as yoga or *Tai Chi*; and, finally, massages to help you achieve that mind-body-spirit integration.

"Best of all, good physical fitness rewards you and enriches your life in ways you wouldn't ordinarily think about. For instance, I wouldn't be able to do all the things I'm doing as a mother, wife, television personality, and worldwide traveler without a great deal of endurance. That endurance would be impossible if I didn't work out regularly."

Your goal is to achieve a high level of physical fitness. How is that defined? With an embarrassment of riches in expertise on fitness, we took to the Internet to see what we could find. We discovered a definition, posted there by Linda Delzeit, that we liked:

- Strength: the ability of muscles to perform work.

- Flexibility: the stretch-capacity and range of motion of the muscles, ligaments, and joint capsules.

- Endurance: the ability to sustain vigorous exercise. This is dependent on good heart and lung functions.

Delzeit suggests four general principles of conditioning:

Overload: working slightly beyond your normal limits.

Progression: always doing just a little bit more.

Regularity: each week three or four aerobic workouts.

Maintenance: based on the rule that it is easier to maintain than to attain. Although it takes about twelve weeks to get fit, it takes only two weeks of doing nothing to get unfit.

Scientists so far haven't completely settled on how much exercise is needed to improve health and prolong longevity. But they do agree that—as with the brain—body exercise is healthful while inactivity is not. In fact, low physical fitness is a powerful predictor of early mortality.

At the Cooper Institute for Aerobics Research in Dallas, Steven N. Blair headed a massive study of more than 25,000 men and 7,000 women. That study provides support for the value of moderate exercise. Blair found that three brisk ten-minute walks a day on most days of the week are as effective as one thirty-minute walk in achieving moderate fitness.

This shift from low to moderate fitness is important, because out-of-shape men and women have about twice the risk of early death compared to more fit and active people. Not only does physical fitness improve one's quality of life, it also protects against heart disease and diabetes. It even provides some protection against high blood pressure, high cholesterol, and smoking, according to many studies.

Menopausal women who exercise regularly—nothing more elaborate than one long walk a week—are 12 percent less likely to die over the next seven years than women who are not physically active. If the activity level is notched up just a bit—bowling, gardening, or walking four or more times per week—that 12 percent figure jumps to 33 percent.

How does exercise confer its health and longevity benefits? At some point, exercise exerts a beneficial effect on the heart and cardiovascular system. Even moderate exercise reduces blood pressure by 6 to 10 mm of mercury (the standard unit measured by a blood pressure cuff). Further, this reduction is maintained for up to thirteen hours.

Cardiologists believe exercise lowers blood pressure by dampening the activity of the sympathetic nervous system. Since enhanced sympathetic tone increases the tension in the walls of arteries, anything that tends to lessen this influence relaxes arterial wall tension and lowers blood pressure. The effect is like replacing a narrow-width hose with one of wider dimension: the water exits under less pressure the wider the hose.

Exercise also increases the volume of blood coursing through the entire vascular system. Long-distance runners have nearly a liter more blood in their vascular systems than is found in the average person. This results from a readjustment in the communication between the heart and the kidneys.

Exercise decreases the sensitivity of a volume control system in the right chamber of the heart, which ordinarily tells the kidneys to remove fluid when the volume increases too much. But with a dampening of the sensitivity of this feedback sensor, the body accommodates for an increase in blood volume.

Among the benefits of expanded blood volume is an increase in the amount of blood pumped with each heartbeat. This increase in efficiency accounts for the lower heart rate of athletes.

An expanded blood volume bestows another benefit. It counteracts the formation of "sludge." Lipids, the villains responsible for arteriosclerosis, are less likely to deposit on blood vessel walls under the more dilute conditions created by an expanded volume.

Exercise reduces the levels of triglyceride fats, the fat component most highly linked with heart attacks. Muscles literally "eat up" any increased fat by creating a special enzyme, lipoprotein lipase (LPL). This enzyme breaks down the triglyceride into smaller components that serve as fuel for the overactive muscles. As an additional benefit, LPL reduces blood cholesterol.

Exercise also strengthens the immune system. As a natural sequence of normal aging, immune function shows an age-related decline. In some cases this can result in a relative immune deficiency and serious dysregulations in immune functioning. Moreover, an already compromised system can be further weakened by mental stress, undernourishment, quick weight loss, and improper hygiene. But whatever the causes, immune system changes can have serious consequences, since we are dependent on our immune system to fight off infections.

Regular moderate physical activity can reverse many of these falloffs in immune functioning. The emphasis here is on *moderate* exercise. Too much exercise and the benefits actually reverse.

"Both chronic stress and unusually heavy chronic exercise can negatively impact immune status," according to a 1997 report by sports medicine specialists at West Virginia University and published by the *International Journal of Sports Medicine.*

Athletes, coaches, and sports doctors have known for years that athletes are especially susceptible during intensive training to infectious illnesses such as upper respiratory infections. This is because chronic intensive exercise—in contrast to moderate exercise—leads to a worsening of immune function.

Exercise also provides orthopedic benefits: fewer falls and subsequent hip and other fractures. As we get older we are much more prone to losing our balance. This is normal and doesn't imply nervous system disease.

Loss of balance results from an increase in the importance with aging of what neurologists refer to as "the proprioceptive sense." Consider what happens when you close your eyes while shampooing in the shower, or take a few steps into a darkened room. At such times your cues about your bodily position in space come from impulses generated from nerves in your legs. These impulses enter the spinal cord, where they are conveyed up to parts of the brain that monitor balance and the position of the parts of your body in space. This is proprioception. As we age, our body seems to depend more on proprioception—in fact, even more so than vision. That's why an older person may fall even when he or she can see clearly everything on the ground and in the environment.

But something can be done about this tendency as we get older for proprioception to outweigh vision. We can practice exercises that enhance balance. The ancient Asian exercise of *Tai Chi* is an excellent choice because it improves the functioning of the balance centers, principally the cerebellum, while it strengthens the thigh muscles, thus increasing one's sense of being firmly grounded and stable. Under such conditions the likelihood of falls decreases tremendously.

With so many obvious health benefits, why don't we all exercise more? Because too many of us hold outmoded ideas about how much exercise is needed. Don't fall into the trap of thinking that exercise is an all-or-nothing phenomenon: either you work out in a gym several times a week or you do nothing. A future centenarian is often going to be too busy for regular attendance at a gym and therefore needs to acquire activity patterns that work almost as well as regular gym attendance.

Listen to what Hildegarde Mahoney said—not yesterday, but several years ago in a *Vogue* magazine interview: "First you have to find the exercise, or the sport, you like. That's half the battle, because it's no use trying to follow anything that bores you or you really have no time for . . . the only way it works is to program exercise into your day. Making a date with yourself, *for* yourself." And Hillie knew what she was talking about: at the time, she was fully booked in far-flung community service—as the wives of corporate heads traditionally were—a hostess and mother of four.

The most recent data to bear out the benefits of exercise are findings from the Cooper Institute for Aerobic Research in Dallas. These show that changes in "lifestyle activity" can provide health benefits equal to a gym-based workout program. Called Project Active, the study compared two groups of sedentary men and women.

Half the participants started working out in a gym for thirty minutes at least three times per week, while the other group integrated exercise routines into their daily lives. At the end of six months, both groups showed similar improvements in such health measures as blood pressure, cholesterol, and general body composition. Best of all, the exercise program of the second group didn't involve anything more elaborate than walking.

Andrea Dunn, director for Project Active, thinks that the best approach is to start by noting in a diary the amount of time you spend sitting each day and then to start chipping away at that block of inactivity. She suggests finding opportunities to take five or six five-minute walks every day. If you want to be really scientific about the process, you can buy a pedometer and try to add 8,000 to 10,000 more steps every day.

Be on the alert for opportunities to walk while at work. Pass up the elevator and walk anything less than three floors; take regular breaks for five-minute walks; in good weather, park your car at the far end of the lot and walk the extra distance.

Walking combined with sound nutritional habits may be all

you need if you're younger than fifty. But if you're older, walking may not be enough, and another form of exercise, weight lifting—or more accurately, weight handling—may be needed. That's because reducing calories also reduces the body's metabolic rate, already diminished in those over fifty. And when you reduce calories the body tries to hold on to fat stores and, in the process, breaks down lean tissue mass. This translates into a loss of muscle and bone.

In sedentary older adults muscle mass declines by about 15 percent between thirty and eighty years of age. This decrease in muscle mass increases the risk of falls and other injuries: the legs simply aren't strong enough to provide firm support. Less muscle mass also leads to obesity (thanks to the body's conserving fat), sugar intolerance or outright diabetes, and impairments in the body's ability to regulate temperature. And since less muscle mass translates into weaker muscle contractions, the skeletal structure is also weakened—a major cause of brittle bones and fractures.

The good news is that this scenario can be reversed, or at least held in check. Even sedentary older people can improve their cardiac function *regardless* of prior physical conditioning, according to research by the National Institute on Aging Gerontology Research Center, the Johns Hopkins Medical Institutions, and the Veterans Administration Center in Baltimore. ". . . [A] novel aspect of this study found that the relative benefits were the same regardless of how fit they were when they started exercising," says Edward Lakatta, chief of the laboratory of cardiovascular science at the National Institute on Aging. This increase in cardiovascular fitness translates into a longer, healthier life.

The secret is a regular program of strength-enhancing exercises using graded weights. Start these exercises in your forties and continue for the rest of your life.

We're not talking here about hefting huge barbells. Rather, pick a weight you can raise and lower between ten and fifteen times without excessive strain or fatigue—just heavy enough to provide the challenge of some gentle strengthening. Five pounds is a good starting weight for most people. Then go on to ten pounds.

The most important thing is not the weight but the repetitions; not the lifting, but the handling; the goal is to increase the number of repetitions rather than to increase the amount of weight lifted. Concentrate on the muscles of the shoulders, arms, calves, and thighs. Finally, give your muscles a chance to recover; restrict the sessions to no more than three times a week.

The key point to remember is that the best weight loss program involves replacing fat with muscle rather than restricting calories. If you combine the walking exercises mentioned above with a sensible weight-handling program, you can keep your weight down; maintain a firm, well-proportioned body; and avoid the dangers accompanying caloric restriction. Best of all, this simple but effective exercise program can easily be accommodated within the time constraints of the busy future centenarian.

If you want a practical and uncomplicated guide to increasing your physical activity, refer to the Activity Pyramid on the next page. This is the creation of Jane Norstrom, manager of health education services for HealthSystem Minnesota. She designed the pyramid in response to the confusion many people expressed to her about how much exercise is sufficient.

Thirty minutes a day of moderate activity is now believed to exert a measurable effect on heart disease, stroke, diabetes, osteoporosis—and depression. The Activity Pyramid is intended as a visual guide on how to integrate these new findings into a practical exercise program. It is modeled on the U.S. Department of Agriculture's Food Guide Pyramid (see Chapter 27),

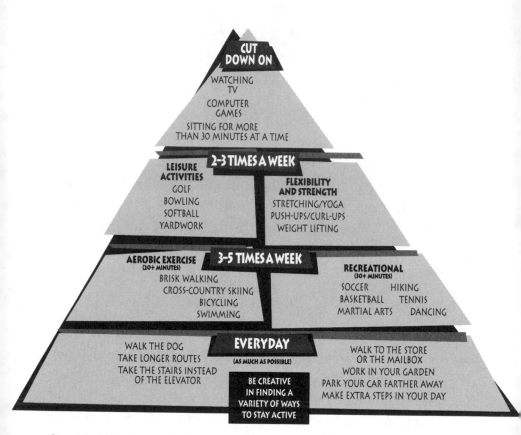

CUT
DOWN ON
WATCHING
TV
COMPUTER
GAMES
SITTING FOR MORE
THAN 30 MINUTES AT A TIME

2–3 TIMES A WEEK

LEISURE
ACTIVITIES
GOLF
BOWLING
SOFTBALL
YARDWORK

FLEXIBILITY
AND STRENGTH
STRETCHING/YOGA
PUSH-UPS/CURL-UPS
WEIGHT LIFTING

AEROBIC EXERCISE
(20+ MINUTES)   3–5 TIMES A WEEK
BRISK WALKING
CROSS-COUNTRY SKIING
BICYCLING
SWIMMING

RECREATIONAL
(30+ MINUTES)
SOCCER   HIKING
BASKETBALL   TENNIS
MARTIAL ARTS   DANCING

EVERYDAY
(AS MUCH AS POSSIBLE)

WALK THE DOG
TAKE LONGER ROUTES
TAKE THE STAIRS INSTEAD
OF THE ELEVATOR

BE CREATIVE
IN FINDING A
VARIETY OF WAYS
TO STAY ACTIVE

WALK TO THE STORE
OR THE MAILBOX
WORK IN YOUR GARDEN
PARK YOUR CAR FARTHER AWAY
MAKE EXTRA STEPS IN YOUR DAY

Copyright ©1996 Institute for Research and Education HealthSystem Minnesota

which emphasizes healthy food choices. The Activity Pyramid emphasizes healthy activity choices.

And last but not least, exercise helps you "keep all your marbles": findings by Marilyn Albert, the Harvard Medical School professor and director of gerontology research at Massachusetts General Hospital, show that exercise produces memory improvement, even in very elderly people.

In short, it is never too late to start. The right time to begin exercising is *now*.

CHAPTER 27

E*at for tomorrow. Establish eating habits that will hold you in good stead for the rest of your life.*

IF YOU WANT AN EASY WAY to remember the value of careful eating, recall the words of the legendary Negro baseball leagues and Hall of Fame pitcher Satchel Paige: "I never eat fatty foods; they angry up the blood."

Famed heart surgeon Michael DeBakey takes his own advice when it comes to avoiding the known health risks for illness. "I have always tried to do this by eating a moderate diet with emphasis on seasonal fruits and vegetables; exercising regularly by walking, climbing stairs, and otherwise incorporating physical activity in my daily routine; pursuing a vigorous schedule of daily activities; and avoiding smoking, excessive alcohol, and other drugs."

Among the factors mentioned by DeBakey, none is more important than diet. Dietary factors are associated with five of the leading ten causes of death: coronary heart disease, certain types of cancer, stroke, non-insulin-dependent diabetes, and atherosclerosis.

A sensible diet even makes sense from the fiscal point of view: 30 percent of national health care expenditures are related to inappropriate diet.

Yet despite the acknowledged wisdom of eating a good diet, few people seem to be practicing that wisdom. Nationwide, ham sandwiches and pizza are the most popular lunch or dinner entrées. We Americans consume more cheese, sugar, and soft drinks per capita than ever. Those of us on diets don't do any better: When the *Washington Post* in February 1997 surveyed the eating habits of 2,617 self-selected volunteers, the paper found that people who drink Ultra Slim-Fast shakes for meals invariably eat candy or other sweets for snacks.

The *Post* asked its readers to "keep track of everything you eat and drink today and send your diary back to us." The responses were interesting. If they were truly representative of our nation's eating habits, all of us, dietwise, would be well on our way toward centenarianism.

Post respondents tended to eat less meat, pizza, fast food, and more fruit, bagels, and turkey sandwiches. So who is consuming all of that sugar, cheese, and soft drinks? The nonresponders: all of those *Post* readers who out of denial or embarrassment failed to submit their diet diary for the day.

"Clearly, the respondents of our survey are not typical. We heard mostly from people (lots of women over forty-five) who wanted to tell somebody—anybody—how healthfully they eat," wrote health reporter Carole Sugarman.

In addition to the self-selected group of *Post* readers, 165 students from three local high schools kept a food diary as part of a classroom assignment. Their responses, unfortunately, were more consistent with our national consumption patterns. Pizza, soda, spaghetti, hamburgers, and french fries were the most common food selections. Overall, the students' diets lacked variety and were deficient in fruits and milk. Will this unhealthy eating pattern persist into adulthood? Several factors increase the likelihood of this happening.

If you're more than thirty years old, your parents probably played a major role in what you ate as a child. Breakfast and dinner were at home, and the food was preselected for you by your parents. Many schools, public and private, had lunch programs that, although far from nutritionally optimal, certainly provided more nutritious fare than what's available today from vending machines, fast-food outlets, and other quick and easy hunger solutions. Most of these changes, of course, are related more to social trends than to strictly dietary issues.

Today there are more single-parent households and working mothers who simply aren't available to influence what their children eat. The regular sit-down dinner that included the whole family has become a thing of the past. In many contemporary American households, parents and children alike wander into the kitchen at odd times, prepare something for themselves out of whatever happens to be lying around, and then eat alone. As a result of these social changes, this is the first generation of children in our nation's history forced to make their own, often unenlightened, choices about their diets.

So what do you tell a preteenager or teenager about diet so that he or she has a fighting chance to make it to 100 years of age? Nutritionists are consistent on this question and, better yet, their recommendations are easy to understand and adhere to.

Decrease dietary fat, lower caloric intake, and eat more fruits and vegetables. Nuts, berries, fruits, and greens should be the dietary foundation, with chicken and fish eaten in moderation according to personal preference. Although red meat doesn't have to be completely eliminated, steaks should be consumed on "special occasions" when there is something to celebrate. Salt, fat, and calories should be limited to prevent weight gain.

Supplements

In addition to a good diet, the Longevity Strategy emphasizes supplements. The best advice at this point is a daily combination of antioxidants (such as vitamins C and E, beta-carotene, selenium) as well as folate and calcium. Keep up supplements of vitamin E, since this vitamin is now known to exert an effect on brain function.

If Alzheimer's patients are given 2,000 International Units (IUs) of vitamin E daily, the illness can be significantly slowed down. Those patients taking vitamin E supplements show a six- to seven-month delay in decline due to the disease, compared to patients not given vitamin E pills. This level of 2,000 IUs, incidentally, is considered the threshold level for side effects with

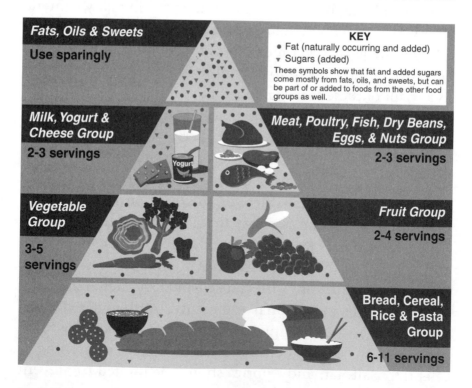

Adapted by Leigh Coriale Design and Illustration. Source: USDA.

the nutrient. That threshold level may be even lower for people taking anticlotting drugs, since vitamin E influences blood-clotting mechanisms and may increase bleeding-type strokes. In other words, a doctor should be consulted before one starts the regular intake of 2,000 IUs a day.

At lower doses, vitamin E exerts other important health influences. Moderate amounts of supplemental vitamin E boost the immune system in people older than sixty-five, according to scientists from the USDA Human Nutrition Research Center on Aging at Tufts University in Boston. They found that a single 200-mg capsule of vitamin E increased T-cell function by 65 percent. The supplement also boosted the level of protection conferred on the body by vaccines. As a secondary bonus, vitamin E is also believed to provide protection from heart disease and cancer.

Although vitamin E is found in high-fat foods such as soybeans, uncooked oils such as vegetable oils and margarine, wheat germ, nuts, and seeds, the amount discovered to be beneficial in the Tufts study (200 mg, with 1 mg roughly equal to 1 IU of vitamin E) cannot be comfortably eaten in a regular diet. The diet must be supplemented with vitamin pills.

One important caveat when it comes to vitamins and other supplements: Dietary recommendations are now under revision. Recommended daily allowances are undergoing update, expansion, and reshaping to include new categories. This revision, the first since 1989, is so extensive that it is being done in seven stages and will not be finished until the year 2000.

As the first of these revisions, the National Academy of Sciences issued new recommendations in August 1997 for five nutrients (calcium, vitamin D, phosphorus, magnesium, and fluoride). In deference to the new expanded demographics, the academy also created two new age categories (fifty-one to seventy, and seventy or older, rather than the previous category that stopped with fifty-one or older).

Hormones

Not only vitamins but also hormone supplements can benefit brain functioning and general health. This is especially true for women. For women past menopause, powerful benefits can be produced via the addition of the female sex hormone estrogen. The hormone affects more than just reproduction and sexual behavior; the hormone also improves memory in normal, healthy women. It is also believed to reduce the risk of Alzheimer's disease and other dementias.

The first hint of the importance of estrogen evolved from the work of Bruce McEwen at Rockefeller University in New York. McEwen surgically removed the ovaries from female rats and then gave them estrogen. He then found an increase in an enzyme, choline acetyltransferase (ChAT), in certain neurons in a part of the brain (the basal forebrain) later discovered to be linked with brain areas (the hippocampus and cerebral cortex) associated with learning and memory.

Estrogen works within the brain by several mechanisms. It helps maintain synapses, the functional contacts between neurons; it cooperates with neurotrophins, a family of molecules that promote the growth and survival of several different classes of neurons; it protects brain cells by acting as an antioxidant, neutralizing the highly reactive free radicals that kill neurons by disintegrating their membranes.

These estrogen effects at the molecular and cellular levels have practical implications. High blood levels of estrogen in rats and monkeys lead to superior performance in memory tasks involving the hippocampus.

Similar mental benefits have been noted in humans. Estrogen given to young women improves their verbal memory. Among postmenopausal women, estrogen therapy reduces the risk of Alzheimer's disease by about 50 percent, according to a study released in June 1997 by scientists participating in the Baltimore Longitudinal Study of Aging.

During the sixteen-year Baltimore study of 472 menopausal or postmenopausal women, estrogen therapy provided a protective effect against dementia. Moreover, it didn't make any difference how long the women had been on estrogen: everybody who took the hormone replacement benefited. In fact, it's never too late to start taking estrogen. The hormone even works in women in the early stages of Alzheimer's disease. It doesn't cure the disease, but it does slow its progression.

Scientists are now enthusiastically searching for new estrogenlike drugs that benefit brain function without risking the development of cancers of the uterus, breast, or ovaries.

Can men benefit from estrogen? Yes, if drugs can be designed that don't lead to increases in breast size, change in body contours, and other feminization effects. Dr. Claudia Kawas, director of the Baltimore study, says, " 'Designer' estrogen, drugs that are currently being developed by a number of pharmaceutical companies, could minimize estrogen's feminizing and other unwanted side effects and provide a potent strategy for both men and women in delaying or reducing death due to Alzheimer's disease in a large segment of the aging population."

The odds are that, in the next five years, estrogen will become a standard supplement to maintain and perhaps even improve mental functioning in both women and men.

Estrogen may also prove to be a preventive for stroke. Stroke and stroke-related brain diseases are the third leading cause of death in the United States (exceeded only by heart disease and cancer). Stroke is the largest single cause of neurologic disability and a major cause of late-life dementia that affects Americans who live into their sixties or beyond.

At the moment, a major long-term trial is under way involving more than 600 postmenopausal women. The Women's Estrogen for Stroke Trial (WEST) aims at determining if estrogen therapy reduces the risk of death or disability from stroke in women past menopause. When the study is completed, it's a good bet that estrogen will prove helpful, as it has in earlier, less extensive trials, in lowering the chances that a post-menopausal woman will suffer a stroke.

CHAPTER 28

Start your longevity program now, and do it one small step at a time.

PROFESSOR MIKE DORIZAS, one of David's professors at the Wharton School of Business at the University of Pennsylvania, taught his students the importance of what he called the Law of the Least Noted Difference, or LND.

Mike used an analogy to make his point. If you put a frog in a pan of steaming hot water, it will immediately attempt to get out. But if you put it in tepid water and then heat that water very, very slowly, you'll boil the frog to death. That's because the frog isn't attuned to subtle and incremental temperature changes. It dies because of its failure to appreciate and respond to the least notable difference in its environment from moment to moment.

In many ways we're like that frog. Certainly, we notice that thirty-pound weight gain when we look at pictures of ourselves taken two years apart. But few of us attend to the weekly half-pound weight gains that, added together over the previous months, account for our added girth.

Most changes in our lives happen like that weight gain. They occur slowly enough that, unless we remain perceptive and observant, they'll remain outside of our awareness. That's why we have to learn to appreciate the least notable differences occurring in every aspect of our lives. This is particularly important when it comes to self-improvement.

The hardest part of any self-improvement program is getting started. Arthur Ashe had a solution for how to get started, paraphrasing Teddy Roosevelt's advice: "To achieve greatness: start where you are, use what you have, do what you can."

The second-hardest part is trying to do it all and then giving up in the face of the inevitable failure that comes when you attempt to undo a lifetime of bad habits overnight.

Get started right now—that takes care of the hardest part. Avoid the physically and emotionally draining experience of the second-hardest part by following the Rule of Ten, which is based on making the Law of the Least Noted Difference work for you.

The Rule of Ten

Each month for the next six months, introduce a 10 percent modification in the following areas of your life.

1. A 10 percent increase in your physical activity. If you exercise two hours a week, twelve minutes more won't be noticed. After only a couple of 10 percent increases you'll be firmly in the zone of optimal exercise and activity.

2. A 10 percent increase in dietary complex carbohydrates (grains, including bread, cereal, and pasta)

3. A 10 percent increase in fiber intake

4. A 10 percent decrease in calories

5. A 10 percent decrease in fat intake

6. A 10 percent increase in sleep and/or naps

7. A 10 percent decrease in alcohol intake (no more than 2–3oz. per day maximum)

8. A 10 percent decrease in stress via use of meditation or any other method that enables you to gain a "this, too, shall pass" perspective; list the ten most stressful things in your life that are destroying your health, and eliminate them one at a time.

9. A 10 percent increase in reading and other mind-expanding, intellectually stimulating activities

10. A 10 percent decrease in tobacco use

Of the ten factors where the goal is slow, incremental reduction, only the last (tobacco) should be continued indefinitely until you reach ground zero. The others should be halted after a few months when an optimal level is achieved. This will vary from person to person. Obviously you don't want to reduce your caloric and fat intake below a certain point. Consultation with a doctor knowledgeable about physical activity and your own health is the best way to go.

The most important decision is deciding to change. Dr. James Prochaska, of the Cancer Prevention Research Consortium at the University of Rhode Island, says that people routinely go through five stages as they make important changes in their lives.

Precontemplation. This stage can last for years. It involves a vague, gnawing awareness of the negative aspects of certain behaviors. For instance, a smoker does not deny that cigarettes cause lung cancer. But he or she doesn't think of it in personal terms: it's always going to involve somebody else. If smoking cessation is thought about at all, it is only a peripheral concern.

Contemplation. This is when the person toys with the idea

of changing. An informational cost-benefit analysis goes on in the person's mind: how hard will it be for me to change, and what are the possible consequences if I don't make the effort? This stage can go on for a long time. In one study of smokers, most remained in this stage for two years.

Preparation. In this stage the person has finally elected to take action. Specific steps are decided upon. Although this is a major step forward, the person is far from being home free. Many have unsuccessfully taken actions in the past year that did not work.

Action. This occurs when actual behaviors are undertaken to change the unwanted behavior. The action phase can range from days to months. People in this stage feel once again in control of their lives while still usually needing help from others.

Maintenance. The prevention of relapse is handled in this stage. It begins six months after first taking action and, depending on the behavior being modified, may last a lifetime.

Understanding these stages is a great help in determining the likelihood of bringing about the desired change in behavior. At each stage, positive reinforcements—rewards—are more effective than punishments.

As adman Bruce Barton put it: "When you're through changing, you're through."

CHAPTER 29

Think of the possibilities. Why stop at 100? Why can't humans live forever?

ONCE YOU GET PROFICIENT at working the Longevity Strategy, you could start thinking of biblical extremes of longevity. But remember, as Ira Gershwin wrote in *Porgy and Bess:* "Methusaleh lived 900 years. But who calls that livin', when no gal will give in, to no one who's 900 years?"

However long any of us may live, nobody wants to spend his or her last years of life sick or disabled. And gerontologists, experts on healthy aging, are changing their thinking about longevity. They're now balancing their efforts at coming up with ways of prolonging life with an equally intense interest in fending off diseases and disabilities and staying healthy as long as possible.

One of the best recent examples of this emphasis on quality of life over quantity has been progress in anti-impotence drugs for men. At least a dozen promising approaches—from pills to injections—are awaiting approval by the U.S. Food and Drug Administration. These remedies offer men and their mates hope of a normal life after illness, but equally important, they will contribute to men's overall longevity by erasing the destructive sense of "losing it" that impotence fosters.

While life expectancy has increased over the past seven decades from forty-seven years to more than seventy-five, so, too, have atherosclerosis (the deposition of fatty material in the lining of the arteries), cancer, heart disease, arthritis, and other diseases. But while these diseases have contributed significantly to increased disability, their role in determining mortality is more ambiguous. If we could make all of them disappear overnight, the average life span would surely increase, but only up to a point.

The smoking and drinking rates in Utah, for instance, are far below the national average. And while the people there enjoy better health, they do not live forever. In fact, they don't live any longer, on average, than people in other parts of the United States. While lifestyle modifications improve health, they do not result in unlimited extensions of the life span. As discussed in chapter 1 on programmed senescence versus the "wear and tear" models of aging, there seems to be an upper limit to just how long we humans can live.

Of course, decreases in illness result in longevity benefits: healthier people are by definition freer of diseases and live longer than sick people do. For proof we have only to look at the increase in life span in the twentieth century. As the level of health care increased, the numbers of people killed by acute illnesses (mostly infections) decreased. In many chronic diseases, the period from the onset to death has been lengthened. The question is whether the life span can be increased indefinitely as a result of lifestyle changes. There is a good reason for doubting the possibility of indefinitely postponing death.

It is not our intention to advocate some misty fantasy of achieving immortality here on Earth. Death is part of the life cycle, and all of us must come to terms with it in our own way. But we do think that good health and longevity to 100 years can be achieved by using the knowledge we now possess. Ours is the most informed generation in history when it comes to health and longevity enhancers. All we have to do is discipline ourselves to apply that knowledge.

Despite the fact that we can't live forever, we will be able to prolong the years of healthful and mindful living. By delaying the age of onset of the first serious chronic disease, years of healthy life are gained. And all the scientific opinion is on the side of prolonged *health* as a more achievable goal than dramatic increases in life span.

The key insight: indefinite postponement of disability— mental and physical—is an achievable goal. By increasing the years of healthy living, we stand a good chance, based on the number of centenarians now living and the many more expected to reach that age over the next quarter century, of becoming centenarians ourselves. More than that, nobody can promise. So far no documented person in the history of the human race has made it beyond 122 years. Will that figure change thanks to some presently unforeseen scientific breakthrough? At the moment that question remains tantalizingly intriguing but unanswerable. We think the answer is yes—but we're optimists.

The Longevity Strategy is not directed toward living indefinitely, nor even toward breaking that record of 122 years. It is directed toward 100 years of healthy living, and that is an achievable goal for you.

CHAPTER 30

D on't wait for a "magic bullet." There is no such thing as a fountain of youth. Despite the promise of genetic research and other potential biological extenders of longevity, don't neglect proven aids to living longer. Don't be fooled into thinking longevity can be found in a bottle.

SCIENTISTS AREN'T REALLY SURE just what aging is. One thing is agreed on, however: aging is not a disease. You are going to get older. "I doubt that aging can be reversed," says Leonard Hayflick, a University of California at San Francisco expert on aging. "That's because aging is the result of changes occurring in molecules and the absence of perfect repair processes. Everything in the universe ages."

The Longevity Strategy doesn't include some kind of mystic belief that aging can be stopped and we will all live forever. But aging can be slowed, and the average life span can and will be significantly lengthened. These advances will come about principally through incorporating into your daily routines the lifestyle changes that are emphasized in this book. In the meantime, read with a hefty dose of skepticism many of the claims now being made for longevity enhancers.

Antiaging panaceas usually involve so-called rejuvenating hormones. The search for rejuvenating hormones can be traced back at least to the Middle Ages, when the blood of young men was infused into old men in anticipation that their long-lost youth could be regained. All that resulted were sometimes fatal transfusion reactions. With the passage of time the emphasis switched from blood to hormones.

In Arthur Conan Doyle's *The Creeping Man,* an aging professor attempts to rejuvenate his libido through the injection of an extract of monkey testicles. While the remedy works, it has an unforeseen side effect: the professor turns into an ape. Today the specter of Doyle's ape-professor is more than just the stuff of fiction. Every hormone carries with it some risk. Included among the hormones enjoying current popularity is melatonin, a product of the pineal gland in the brain. While melatonin is helpful in the management of jet lag and some forms of insomnia, its life-extending qualities are pure conjecture. In addition, the beneficial effects in animals may carry unwanted and unacceptable risks in humans.

"Through the use of melatonin it is possible to increase life span in animals. In some cases this price is rather disproportionate to profit—some pathological processes could develop, including cancer," according to Vladimir N. Anisimov of the N. N. Petrov Research Institute of Oncology in St. Petersburg, Russia.

Another supplemental hormone with an enthusiastic following is DHEA, sometimes referred to as the "mother hormone" because the body converts it into the sex hormones estrogen and testosterone. Recently DHEA has been labeled a "biomarker for age," since from youth through early adulthood the adrenal gland secretes the hormone in steadily rising quantities. At that point, somewhere in the early twenties, the output begins to taper. By age eighty, people have 80 to 90 percent less DHEA in their blood than they had at age twenty-five.

The decline in DHEA with advancing age has spurred this question: if body deterioration accompanies the decline of DHEA and other hormones, could aging be reversed or at least held at bay if these hormones are replaced? Hidden in this question is an unproved assumption. Just because a hormone level drops with increasing aging, it doesn't necessarily follow that hormones cause aging or that providing supplements will prolong life.

In addition, DHEA and other hormones exert powerful and unwanted effects in the body. In men DHEA may stimulate the growth of prostate cancer. Women taking DHEA risk scalp hair loss, deepening of the voice, and an increase in bodily hair growth.

"The scary thing about something like DHEA is that it could circulate and be converted to estrogen or testosterone—which could be exactly what a tumor needs to grow," according to Richard Sprott, director of the biology of aging programs at the National Institute on Aging.

Even the use of antioxidants involves certain assumptions that we believe are reasonable yet, to be fair, remain incompletely proven.

"There's no evidence that taking antioxidants actually results directly in the tying up of free radicals that would otherwise do damage," according to Leonard Hayflick. "It's simply assumed that if you ingest lots of vitamin C it will get to the right places in your body to prevent free radical damage."

Despite these caveats, we suggest the use of antioxidants. The evidence for their effectiveness, although not overwhelmingly convincing, remains strikingly impressive. It's likely that the officially recommended daily allowances will, like the dietary recommendation for calcium, be increased by a significant amount. But until we know for sure the optimal amounts of each vitamin, it's best to take them at no more than twice the recommended daily allowances. Avoid ingesting amounts that may prove toxic.

Is fish "brain food"? Controversy exists in regard to the ingestion of chemical precursors for some of the neurotransmitters. Only a few years ago some dietitians were suggesting that we eat a lot of fish. This nutritional nostrum was based on the fact that fish contain high concentrations of choline, a precursor for acetylcholine, the neurotransmitter important in memory and other brain functions. But when doctors radioactively tagged some ingested choline and tried to detect its signal using brain imaging, they failed to turn up convincing evidence that a significant amount of the choline wound up in the brain. Besides, the chemical precursor must do more than just enter the brain. It also must be incorporated into the metabolic cycles that underlie the brain's operation. The situation is similar to bringing electrical supplies to the site of a power failure. Physical proximity isn't enough; everything must be "hooked up" in way that guarantees normal functioning.

In addition, it's unlikely that the brain, with its hundreds if not thousands of neurotransmitters and bioactive chemicals, will be significantly altered in its functioning by an adjustment in a single component of its vast chemical repertory. The situation is similar to trying to bring about an improvement in a symphony orchestra by concentrating on only one instrument:

while sour notes played on a single instrument can unnerve a whole orchestra, it's unlikely that an improved performance by only one instrument will bring about vast improvements in the performance of the entire orchestra.

At this point it's wisest to be cautious about the use of certain dietary supplements. Within the next year or so expect to hear a lot more about what does and doesn't make sense. By the year 2000 the National Academy of Sciences' seven-stage revision of the RDAs (recommended daily allowances) will be completed. Don't be surprised if there are major changes in the RDAs. When the National Academy scientists in August 1997 recommended decreasing the RDA of vitamin D, it was the first time that scientists acknowledged publicly that some nutrients can be unsafe at too-high levels. Our best advice under these circumstances? Keep abreast of what's being published about nutrition, and take your cues from scientific research and not from the hype generated by health food outlets that have a financial interest in urging you to ingest large amounts of supplements in higher-than-recommended or higher-than-necessary doses.

CHAPTER 31

K*eep up with research. Almost daily, scientific research is turning up findings relevant to longevity. It may well find application in your own lifetime.*

IN SEPTEMBER 1997 Thomas T. Perls, whom we quoted discussing centenarians in chapter 1, published with colleagues at Beth Israel–Deaconess Medical Center in Boston an intriguing report on longevity in women. They compared deceased centenarians to older women who had died in their seventies. They discovered that those women who had given birth in their forties were more likely to live to 100. About 19 percent of the women who had given birth after turning forty lived on to become centenarians, versus just 5.5 percent of the other group.

In reporting that finding in the journal *Nature,* the scientists speculated that later-life pregnancy may be a marker for slow-running biological clocks. Another reason may be that women with later births produced estrogen for a longer time and thus were protected for more years against Alzheimer's disease and heart disease. "By avoiding, or at least delaying, diseases associated with aging that can cause premature mortality such as Alzheimer's disease, heart disease, or stroke, these women [who have a prolonged exposure to estrogen] can therefore achieve greater longevity," the scientists concluded. Perhaps this might find practical application as more women forty years or older seek to become pregnant and the double reward of a late-life baby coupled with a greater chance of living to 100.

A more complete understanding of longevity will require greater knowledge of the molecular biology underlying the aging process. For instance, scientists have known for years that lowering an animal's caloric intake not only lowers metabolism but also can cause that animal to live longer. This is true across a broad range of animal species, extending from worms to mice and rats. One wag suggested to us that this "rate of living" theory provides a perfect excuse for inactivity in the pursuit of longevity.

But seriously, is it likely that caloric restriction can extend our life span? So far the work on rhesus monkeys hasn't gone on long enough to decide that question. In creatures like ourselves it's even harder to decide, because we live so long. A 20 percent increase in longevity would require an observation period of more than 100 years. Besides, how many people would be willing to live their entire lives on a calorically restricted diet?

At this point the value of serious caloric restriction in humans remains controversial. Scientists do agree, however, that future genetic discoveries may provide the means to significantly extend human life. In an interview with the *New York Times,* Dr. Caleb E. Finch, a world-recognized longevity researcher at the University of Southern California, expressed his confidence that the human life span can be increased when scientists learn more about genes.

"As we learn more about the specific behavior of genes . . . we will be able to modify many aspects of aging," says Dr. Finch, who suggests the existence of ". . . fundamental mechanisms that prevail among all multicellular organisms that may be very informative in managing human aging."

Cloning is another scientific advance with great potential for modifying and extending the human life span. Dolly, the sheep grown from an egg containing inserted DNA from the breast tissue of a six-year-old ewe, is living proof that, at least in sheep, fully mature cells taken from anywhere in the body can be reprogrammed. Thus skin cells or liver cells—indeed, cells from anywhere in the body—can be induced to produce the whole organism. While cloning of a human is ethically unacceptable, other human applications are likely. Doctors will soon be able to remove a small amount of normal tissue from a patient and then reprogram the cells to differentiate into a specific kind of cell—bone, for instance, or skin or muscle. When the transformation is complete, the tissue could then be grafted into the patient. This could be done without fear of rejection, since the patient's immune system would recognize the new tissue as "self."

At the moment, scientists are trying to develop reprogramming techniques to replace damaged or aging cells with younger cells in organs throughout the body. For instance, a simple white blood cell might be taken from a child and stored for future replacement organs as the child aged. So far such goals have proved elusive. Nevertheless, the research is actively under way, and all of us may have available in the not-so-distant future the means of living longer via genetic manipulation.

Only a few years ago, such a possibility of greater longevity seemed more like something from a science-fiction novel than from a mainstream science report. But that's how science has always worked: one generation's wildest fantasies become the next generation's everyday technology. Who would have predicted only twenty years ago faxes, e-mail, and a worldwide

Net—much less cloning, imaging, and artificial intelligence? Such prognostications would have been considered evidence of distinct eccentricity if not downright lunacy.

Our ideas about the brain are also changing rapidly. It's not an exaggeration to say that we are in the midst of a conceptual revolution. For instance, traditional wisdom has it that brain cells, neurons, never duplicate themselves, like other body cells, such as those in the liver, the bones, or the skin. As a result, lost brain cells were thought until recently to be irreplaceable. You've probably heard this dire assessment in the form of the aphorism "We lose 50,000 brain cells per day." That dismaying concept is simply wrong.

As mentioned early in this book, neuroscientists now know that extensive neuronal loss isn't normal or inevitable at all in a healthy brain. What's more—and this is the exciting part— recent research indicates that neurons can be regenerated and even replaced. Although this is so far confined to animals and a very limited number of experiments with human Parkinson's disease patients, there is no reason to doubt that similar results will soon be possible in humans.

"Neuronal replacement in the adult is not only possible but might become simple," according to Ronald McKay of the Laboratory of Molecular Biology, National Institute of Neurological Disorders and Stroke. McKay believes that neuronal replacement will be the natural result of new knowledge of how cells differentiate in the brain. Experimental research on early brain development reveals the existence of stem cells, early precursors that can differentiate into neurons or other supporting cells (referred to as *glia,* from the Greek word for glue) in the brain.

When these stem cells are removed from one animal, grown in culture, and then reinserted into the brain of another animal,

they differentiate into healthy neurons. So far this technology
has been limited to the development of treatments for diseases
such as Parkinson's. But there is good reason to believe this technology could be applied to counteracting some of the nerve cell
loss accompanying normal aging.

Neuroscientists are also forging new concepts about the
nature of the neuron. "In some ways neurons are like people,"
according to Carl W. Cotman, director of the Institute for Brain
Aging and Dementia of the University of California at Irvine.
"They have to live with others, and yet have to look out for
themselves, too. Each is slightly different and produces different gene products. This is one of the reasons why neurons do not
all respond the same way to the same experience."

Cotman's recent research on nerve cells reveals that actively
"firing" cells are more resistant to a host of damaging agents.
"That to me is confirmation that active nerve cells have the
capacity to protect themselves," Cotman tells us.

The bottom line: an active "firing" nerve cell is healthier
than one that is inactive. That same principle holds in regard
to the brain as a whole: use it or lose it.

Cotman has also discovered that exercise actually stimulates
brain cells to form more synapses. He compared rats that do no
physical activity to others that were engaged in wheel running.
In the hippocampus and some cortical areas of the active rats,
he found higher levels of a substance, BDNF (brain derived neu-
rotrophic factor), that promotes nerve growth. Only a few days
of voluntary running will induce in the hippocampus almost a
doubling in the expression of BDNF, he found.

When Cotman discussed his findings at an informal discussion at Leisure World, a member of the audience asked a
provocative question: What happens if you're thinking or learning at the same time you're exercising? Does that induce even
more BDNF and synaptic growth?

To find out, Cotman compared rats forced to wend their way through a water maze with other rats swimming the same distance but without the additional demand of the maze. "We found that learning plus the exercise is better in terms of brain stimulation and synapse induction," he said, "than just the exercise alone. It's another illustration that using brain cells helps to maintain them."

Using our neurons also makes them more resistant to harmful agents. If neurons are actively firing, they're able to resist the chemical insults better. "That to me provides confirmation that active brain cells have the capacity to protect themselves and to encode other changes that they are going through," says Cotman.

Neuronal stability in the face of physical challenge is a hopeful finding. We can forget about the cliché that the brain cannot correct itself after injury. Cotman and others are showing that healthy nerve cells grow collateral sprouts and make new synapses to replace those lost. This stabilizes nerve circuits, counteracts additional cell loss, and prevents potentially greater functional decline.

Even in people afflicted with Alzheimer's disease, a robust sprouting reaction occurs in the damaged hippocampal pathways. Cotman and others seek to bolster this self-protective effort by the brain. "Our main goal is to understand the molecular mechanisms underlying brain growth in order to develop new therapies," says Cotman.

But what about the healthy brain, the brain we want to function successfully for more than 100 years? Cotman is convinced that healthy life extension and preserved brain functioning beyond 100 is ". . . definitely doable. The most important contribution, I believe, will come from diet modification."

And it is important that we supplement our diet with vitamin pills, because scientists are moving toward the conclusion that as we get older, the vitamins available from our diets may not be sufficient. Vitamin C may determine the quality of mental functioning in elderly people, according to a study released by the Environmental Epidemiology Unit of the University of Southampton. "A high vitamin C intake may protect against both cognitive impairment and cerebrovascular disease," the investigators concluded. What's more, the doses of vitamins required to maintain optimum brain function may be in excess of what is now recommended.

The take-home message: the brain needs the same vitamins and nutrients as the rest of the body, but *it needs more of them.* Unfortunately, the current minimum daily nutritional requirements do not pay sufficient attention to the brain's unique needs. For one thing, the brain uses more oxygen per unit volume and produces more oxidation products than any other bodily organ. Thus the brain is uniquely susceptible to the damage caused by oxidation reactions.

"Our goal now is to establish another set of optimal requirements to preserve the quality of the aging nervous system and to create greater and greater numbers of healthy centenarians," says Cotman. "Antioxidants will be the chief component of this nutritional strategy; we may need more antioxidants as we age. That's because as we get older we may be more susceptible to the toxic effects of free radicals and oxidants. The brain simply needs more antioxidants at that stage of life. Neurons burn an enormous amount of oxygen."

At the moment the use of antioxidant supplements such as vitamins C and E to promote longevity is supported by a vast amount of research. Areas of legitimate controversy concern how much should be taken and what is the optimal mix that is most likely to be effective. Expect to hear more on these issues of brain health over the next five years. In the meantime, select an antioxidant formulation and take it regularly.

As we've said, expect also that research on degenerative brain diseases over the next decade will contribute significantly to longevity. Until recently, neuroscientists knew little about the dynamic malfunctions that underlie many of the most common brain diseases. Now that is changing fast.

With the prevention of degenerative brain diseases, many of us will have a shot at achieving a healthy and extended life span. Longevity will become a reality for the majority instead of, as in the past, just a small number of unusually lucky people.

CONCLUSION

Enjoy "the last of life, for which the first was made."

THERE YOU HAVE OUR IDEAS about how to achieve a healthy and active fourth quarter. Medical science is giving us the body to blow out 100 candles on our birthday cake; brain scientists are helping us to maintain an active and creative mind. By applying the principles in this book, we believe you can significantly increase your longevity. Nobody can *guarantee* how long any person may live, of course. Longevity isn't an automatic consequence of sensible and healthy living. The unpredictable always lurks in the background. Accidents happen. Life has to be lived on its own terms, and those terms differ for each of us.

During the next decade and beyond, scientists will teach you more about what you can do to lead a longer, healthier life. But to take advantage of this new knowledge, you have to know about it. Keep current, therefore, with scientific advances, particularly new discoveries about the brain. Here are some of the areas in which we expect further breakthroughs on longevity:

Over the next decade, watch for considerable progress in our understanding of how the brain is "wired." This will extend from life *in utero* up to the fully mature brain of the healthy centenarian. This understanding of the brain over the life span will provide clues on such things as how we can continue to learn most efficiently during our later adult years.

Expect new treatments for strokes and spinal cord injury.

Research at the molecular level will be furthered by the Human Genome Project. One of the benefits of this project will be the identification of the genes responsible for schizophrenia and manic-depression, the two most common neuropsychiatric illnesses. Treatment for these illnesses will begin earlier in life, thanks to earlier diagnosis made possible by genetic screening and PET scans or other technological tools.

Within the next decade, scientists will complete the map of the 100,000 human genes strung along the 23 human chromosomes in our cells. This will provide genetic information on each one of us that can be used to anticipate the illnesses we are prone to. Further, these personalized DNA sequences for each person will not require anything more elaborate than a genetic analysis of blood and urine samples. According to the project's director, Francis Collins, "It is reasonably likely that by the year 2010, a printout can be created showing an individual's risks for future diseases based on the genes that person had inherited."

Doctors will be able to use these DNA "blueprints" to predict your mathematical chances of coming down with any number of diseases. Earlier diagnostic and treatment approaches will then result in cure or treatments for diseases that threaten to shorten your life span. The battle will be fought at the level of "molecular medicine"—diseases encountered and conquered at the molecular level. Computer simulations and virtual reality recreations of viruses and bacteria will become standard. Using these high-tech tools, it will be possible for doctors, without laying hands on their patient, to attack these molecular desperadoes at the precise genetic weak points in their molecular armor. All of these measures will increase longevity via the early detection and cure of illnesses that at the moment can kill or disable you.

Look for new brain-based approaches to addictions. Already there is strong evidence of a genetic predisposition to alcoholism and reason to be confident that the gene or genes will soon be identified. In the past five years evidence has accumulated that two brain areas—the "ventral tegmental area" in the brain stem and the nucleus accumbens, part of the emotional regulatory (limbic) system—are involved in addictions. Drugs under development will key in on these important areas. They hold promise for counteracting the effects of addicting drugs. Even if you're not personally involved in addiction, you will benefit in terms of longevity. A society free of addicted individuals is one in which fewer members die prematurely in alcohol- and drug-related accidents and crimes.

More advances will be made in the next decade in understanding and treating Parkinson's, Alzheimer's, and Huntington's diseases. Recently observed cell changes in Huntington's disease are providing an opportunity for the development of drugs that could short-circuit the progress of the disease and perhaps prevent it in people at risk.

At the moment, research in Huntington's is proceeding at a torrid pace, led by Columbia University's Nancy Wexler. The Huntington's gene discovery dates back only four years. Since that discovery, scientists have learned that several other brain disorders follow a similar genetic pattern. Included in these diseases is fragile-X syndrome, the most common cause of mental retardation in our nation. Many brain scientists expect genetic treatments to be available in the not too distant future that will make possible early prenatal diagnosis and, hopefully, treatment.

While Parkinson's and Alzheimer's diseases are distressingly common, Huntington's is fortunately rare. But rare diseases often have a lot to teach us that can be applied to more common disorders. Indeed, widely applicable principles have often been discovered through research on rare diseases. It is likely that drug research aimed at dementia (senile brain disease) from any cause will benefit all of us undergoing normal brain aging. Among the likely benefits will be memory enhancers, mood stabilizers, and perhaps even drugs capable of raising our IQ performances.

Brain research will also shed light on normal thinking and emotional processes. It is now possible using functional brain imaging techniques such as PET scans and functional MRI scans to zero in on those brain areas that are involved in emotions. Additional research will provide a window on brain functioning during everyday mental states although, according to W. Maxwell Cowan, ". . . research is still in an early stage in identifying genes for complex behaviors like disturbed thinking or mood swings."

Brain disorders must remain a national research and fiscal priority. Did you know that we Americans spend $14 billion a year on cut flowers but only $12 billion a year on medical research? America must not go down in history as a society that cared more about our flowers than about our brains. As David observes, "Cut flowers have no roots and die soon, but brain research blooms and is with us at all times."

Fortunately, the brain is no longer the formidable and somewhat forbidding organ it once was. The public knows more now about the brain than has any other generation in history. As a result of this increase in knowledge, we are no longer afraid of the brain, nor do we as often stigmatize, as we once did, those afflicted with brain diseases. In the near future all brain illnesses will be perceived as diseases rather than as character weaknesses. Indeed, it's turning out that brain science is the most enlightening and liberating of disciplines: as we learn more about the brain, we learn more about ourselves. Consciousness is life; for each one of us, *we are our brain.*

The most important longevity-promoting insights will involve not just the brain but also brain-body interaction. When Richard was in medical school, very little time was spent by most teachers in instructing future doctors on the emotional and psychological aspects of health and disease. Part of this reluctance resulted from ignorance: the teachers simply didn't know much about brain-body interactions. Now all that has changed, thanks to discoveries gleaned, in many cases, by researchers carefully observing the connections between illnesses and lifestyle.

As we've said, stress is one of the most important causes of degenerative diseases. Firm evidence exists linking stress to heart attack rates, survival, and post-heart attack depression; survival after bypass heart surgery; survival rates from breast cancer; the incidence of colon cancer; and decreases in the bone density in women, along with higher levels of the stress hormone cortisol.

The discovery that stress is a causative factor in these illnesses has vast treatment implications. It has and will continue to revolutionize how medicine is practiced in the next century. It will also lead to enhanced longevity, since the emphasis will shift from a hierarchy where doctors dispense medicine to largely uninformed patients to a network of professionals trained to educate patients in lifestyle changes that have the potential, in some instances, to make medication unnecessary.

Each of us will be at the center of this new effort: We will take responsibility for making the changes in our lives that will enhance our likelihood of living longer, healthier lives. We will all be learning new, healthy ways of dealing with our anger, our competitiveness, our feelings of loneliness and isolation—all major risk factors for early death and/or disability.

Medicine's search for knowledge will be furthered by advances in physics. These advances will lead to new generations of imaging devices. Soon high-resolution machines will be able to take "pictures" in real time. They will make it possible to identify and localize specific brain functions. For instance, in the past year neuroscientists at Wellcome Department of Cognitive Neurology, Institute of Neurology, London, carried out a PET scan study of the brains of London cabdrivers. PET scans use radioactive glucose to detect activity in the brain (the brain burns glucose, and this consumption is increased in the most active areas; the scanner records the radioactive signal as bright areas while making the image).

By observing what areas of the PET image are brightest, neuroscientists can tell what brain area is most active when a task is carried out. In the case of the cabdrivers, the researchers found that the right hippocampus was activated when the cab drivers mentally recalled complex routes. But this activation did not take place during tasks involving other types of complex memory. For example, when asked to recall the plots of familiar famous films, activation took place in another area (the left frontal lobe) of the brain. Thus the study shows that in humans the ability to remember the route to a destination requires the right hippocampus.

The cabdriver study is only one kind of insight we can expect from applied brain research using imaging devices. Imaging techniques will reveal for us specific and enlightening details about commonalities and differences in healthy brain functioning from one person to another; it will come into greater use to help diagnose brain disorders. Already we know that people with dyslexia, while reading, activate different brain areas from normal readers. This finding establishes dyslexia as a brain-related dysfunction and not a character flaw or "retardation"—another example of the liberating effect of brain research we mentioned earlier.

\#

All in all, it's an exciting time to stay alive. Brain research is poised to bring about the most dramatic enhancement of human longevity in human history. The goal, as summed up by Dr. Ernst Wynder, who cofounded with David the American Health Foundation, is to "help you die young, as late as possible."

Unlike most of the centenarians living today, you, if you make it to 100, will be better able to remember and use what you've learned during your century. Brain science will enable you to do that. Memory-enhancing drugs, just a few short years away, will help you retain more of what you have learned and observed. You will be able, in the poet's words, to enjoy "the last of life, for which the first was made." Your challenge now is the pleasurable one of making sure you live a varied and fulfilling life that will be worth remembering.

A SPECIAL
ACKNOWLEDGMENT
BY DAVID MAHONEY TO
DANA ALLIANCE MEMBERS

THE LONGEVITY STRATEGY is a labor of love and hope, for which I owe a tremendous debt of gratitude to all the members of the Dana Alliance for Brain Initiatives. In their five years of working to help the public understand the promise of brain research, these 173 men and women have inspired and moved me in ways that words are simply inadequate to express. In that sense, this book is theirs even though it is not an Alliance book; it never could have been written without them, their work, their faith, and their optimism. We look forward to even further progress in the future. Thus I would like to acknowledge each member here.

Members of the Dana Alliance
for Brain Initiatives

Bernard W. Agranoff, M.D.
University of Michigan
Ann Arbor, Mich.

Albert J. Aguayo, M.D.
Montreal General Hospital Research
  Institute
Montreal, Canada

Marilyn S. Albert, Ph.D.
Harvard Medical School
Boston, Mass.

Duane F. Alexander, M.D.
National Institute of Child Health
  and Human Development
Bethesda, Md.

Luigi Amaducci, M.D.
University of Florence
Florence, Italy

Nancy C. Andreasen, M.D., Ph.D.
The University of Iowa Hospitals
  and Clinics
Iowa City, Iowa

Arthur K. Asbury, M.D.
University of Pennsylvania School
  of Medicine
Philadelphia, Pa.

Jack D. Barchas, M.D.
Cornell University Medical College
New York, N.Y.

Robert L. Barchi, M.D., Ph.D.
University of Pennsylvania Medical
  Center
Philadelphia, Pa.

Yves-Alain Barde, M.D.
Max-Planck Institute for Psychiatry
Martinsried, Germany

Allan I. Basbaum, Ph.D.
University of California, San
  Francisco
San Francisco, Calif.

Ursula Bellugi, Ed.D.
The Salk Institute for Biological
  Studies
La Jolla, Calif.

Katherine L. Bick, Ph.D.
The Charles A. Dana Foundation
Wilmington, N.C.

Anders Bjorklund, M.D., Ph.D.
University of Lund
Lund, Sweden

Ira B. Black, M.D.
UMDNJ—Robert Wood Johnson
  Medical School
Piscataway, N.J.

Peter McLaren Black, M.D., Ph.D.
Harvard Medical School
Boston, Mass.

Colin Blakemore, Sc.D., D.Sc., F.R.S.
University of Oxford
Oxford, U.K.

Floyd E. Bloom, M.D.
The Scripps Research Institute
La Jolla, Calif.

Monte S. Buchsbaum, M.D.
Mount Sinai School of Medicine
New York, N.Y.

Rosalie A. Burns, M.D.
Allegheny University of the Health
  Sciences
Philadelphia, Pa.

John H. Byrne, Ph.D.
Houston Health Science Center—
  University of Texas
Houston, Tex.

Benjamin S. Carson Sr., M.D.
Johns Hopkins Medical
  Institutions
Baltimore, Md.

William A. Catterall, Ph.D.
University of Washington
Seattle, Wash.

Nicholas G. Cavarocchi
C R Associates
Washington, D.C.

Connie L. Cepko, Ph.D.
Harvard Medical School
Boston, Mass.

Dennis W. Choi, M.D., Ph.D.
Washington University School of
  Medicine
St. Louis, Mo.

Robert C. Collins, M.D.
University of California, Los Angeles
Los Angeles, Calif.

Martha Constantine-Paton, Ph.D.
Yale University
New Haven, Conn.

Robert M. Cook-Deegan, M.D.
National Academy of Sciences
Washington, D.C.

Leon N. Cooper, Ph.D.
Brown University
Providence, R.I.

Carl W. Cotman, Ph.D.
University of California, Irvine
Irvine, Calif.

W. Maxwell Cowan, M.D., Ph.D.
Howard Hughes Medical Institute
Chevy Chase, Md.

Rex W. Cowdry, M.D.
National Institute of Mental Health
Rockville, Md.

Joseph T. Coyle, M.D.
Harvard Medical School
Belmont, Mass.

Antonio Damasio, M.D., Ph.D.
University of Iowa College of
  Medicine
Iowa City, Iowa

Hanna Damasio, M.D.
University of Iowa College of
  Medicine
Iowa City, Iowa

Robert B. Daroff, M.D.
University Hospitals of Cleveland
Cleveland, Ohio

William C. de Groat, Ph.D.
University of Pittsburgh School of
  Medicine
Pittsburgh, Pa.

Martha Bridge Denckla, M.D.
Johns Hopkins University
Baltimore, Md.

Raymond J. DePaulo Jr., M.D.
Johns Hopkins University School of
  Medicine
Baltimore, Md.

David A. Drachman, M.D.
University of Massachusetts Medical
  Center
Worcester, Mass.

Felton Earls, M.D.
Harvard School of Public Health
Boston, Mass.

Gerald M. Edelman, M.D., Ph.D.
The Scripps Research Institute
La Jolla, Calif.

Gerald D. Fischbach, M.D.
Harvard Medical School
Boston, Mass.

Kathleen M. Foley, M.D.
Memorial Sloan-Kettering Cancer
  Center
New York, N.Y.

Ellen Frank, Ph.D.
Western Psychiatric Institute and
  Clinic
Pittsburgh, Pa.

Fred H. Gage, Ph.D.
University of California, San Diego
La Jolla, Calif.

Michael S. Gazzaniga, Ph.D.
Dartmouth College
Hanover, NH

Sid Gilman, M.D.
University of Michigan Medical
  Center
Ann Arbor, Mich.

Patricia S. Goldman-Rakic, Ph.D.
Yale University School of Medicine
New Haven, Conn.

Murray Goldstein, D.O., M.P.H
United Cerebral Palsy Research and
  Education Foundation
Washington, D.C.

Frederick K. Goodwin, M.D.
George Washington University
  Medical Center
Washington, D.C.

Enoch Gordis, M.D.
National Institute on Alcohol Abuse
  and Alcoholism
Bethesda, Md.

Barry Gordon, M.D., Ph.D.
The Johns Hopkins Hospital
Baltimore, Md.

Gary Gottlieb, M.D., M.B.A.
Friends Hospital
Philadelphia, Pa.

Jordan Grafman, Ph.D.
National Institute on Neurological
  Disorders and Stroke
Bethesda, Md.

Bernice Grafstein, Ph.D.
Cornell University Medical College
New York, N.Y.

Ann M. Graybiel, Ph.D.
Massachusetts Institute of
  Technology
Cambridge, Mass.

William T. Greenough, Ph.D.
University of Illinois at Urbana-
  Champaign
Urbana, Il.

Murray Grossman, M.D., Ph.D.
Hospital of the University of
  Pennsylvania
Philadelphia, Pa.

Robert G. Grossman, M.D.
Baylor College of Medicine
Houston, Tex.

Robert J. Gumnit, M.D.
MINCEP Epilepsy Care
Minneapolis, Minn.

James F. Gusella, Ph.D.
Harvard Medical School
Charlestown, Mass.

Zach W. Hall, Ph.D.
National Institute on Neurological
  Disorders and Stroke
Bethesda, Md.

Mary E. Hatten, Ph.D.
The Rockefeller University
New York, N.Y.

Stephen F. Heinemann, Ph.D.
The Salk Institute for Biological
  Studies
San Diego, Calif.

John G. Hildebrand, Ph.D.
University of Arizona
Tucson, Ariz.

Susan Hockfield, Ph.D.
Yale University School of Medicine
New Haven, Conn.

Richard J. Hodes, M.D.
National Institute on Aging
Bethesda, Md.

H. Robert Horvitz, Ph.D.
Massachusetts Institute of
  Technology
Cambridge, Mass.

Chung Y. Hsu, M.D., Ph.D.
Washington University School of
  Medicine
St. Louis, Mo.

David H. Hubel, M.D.
Harvard Medical School
Boston, Mass.

A. J. Hudspeth, M.D., Ph.D.
The Rockefeller University
New York, N.Y.

Steven E. Hyman, M.D.
National Institute of Mental Health
Rockville, Md.

Kay Redfield Jamison, Ph.D.
Johns Hopkins University School of
  Medicine
Washington, D.C.

Richard T. Johnson, M.D.
Johns Hopkins University School of
  Medicine
Baltimore, Md.

Edward G. Jones, M.D., Ph.D.
University of California, Irvine
Irvine, Calif.

Robert J. Joynt, M.D., Ph.D.
University of Rochester
Rochester, N.Y.

Lewis L. Judd, M.D.
University of California, San Diego
La Jolla, Calif.

Eric R. Kandel, M.D.
Columbia University College of
  Physicians and Surgeons
New York, N.Y.

Robert Katzman, M.D.
University of California, San Diego
La Jolla, Calif.

Claudia H. Kawas, M.D.
Johns Hopkins University School of
  Medicine
Baltimore, Md.

Zaven S. Khachaturian, Ph.D.
The Ronald and Nancy Reagan
  Research Institute of the
  Alzheimer's Association
Potomac, Md.

Masakazu Konishi, Ph.D.
California Institute of Technology
Pasadena, Calif.

Michael Kuhar, Ph.D.
Emory University
Atlanta, GA

Anand Kumar, M.D.
University of Pennsylvania School
  of Medicine
Philadelphia, Pa.

Story C. Landis, Ph.D.
National Institute on Neurological
  Disorders and Stroke
Bethesda, Md.

Lynn Therese Landmesser, Ph.D.
Case Western Reserve University
Cleveland, Ohio

Thomas W. Langfitt, M.D. (Ret.)
The Glenmede Corporation
Philadelphia, Pa.

Joseph LeDoux, Ph.D.
New York University
New York, N.Y.

Alan I. Leshner, Ph.D.
National Institute on Drug Abuse
Rockville, Md.

Irwin B. Levitan, Ph.D.
Brandeis University
Waltham, Mass.

Margaret S. Livingstone, Ph.D.
Harvard Medical School
Boston, Mass.

Rodolfo R. Llinas, M.D.
New York University Medical Center
New York, N.Y.

Don M. Long, M.D.
Johns Hopkins University School of
   Medicine
Baltimore, Md.

Peter R. MacLeish, Ph.D.
Morehouse School of Medicine
Atlanta, Ga.

Bertha K. Madras, Ph.D.
Harvard Medical School
Southborough, Mass.

Joseph B. Martin, M.D., Ph.D.
Harvard Medical School
Boston, Mass.

Robert L. Martuza, M.D.
Georgetown University Medical
   Center
Washington, D.C.

Richard Mayeux, M.D., M.S.E.
Columbia University College of
   Physicians and Surgeons
New York, N.Y.

Bruce S. McEwen, Ph.D.
The Rockefeller University
New York, N.Y.

James L. McGaugh, Ph.D.
University of California, Irvine
Irvine, Calif.

Guy M. McKhann, M.D.
Johns Hopkins University
Baltimore, Md.

Michael M. Merzenich, Ph.D.
University of California, San
   Francisco
San Francisco, Calif.

Marek-Marsel Mesulam, M.D.
Northwestern University Medical
   School
Chicago, Il.

Bradie Metheny
Washington Fax
South Dartmouth, Mass.

Brenda A. Milner, Sc.D.
McGill University
Montréal, P. Q., Canada

Richard C. Mohs, Ph.D.
Mount Sinai School of Medicine
Bronx, N.Y.

John H. Morrison, Ph.D.
Mount Sinai School of Medicine
New York, N.Y.

Vernon B. Mountcastle, M.D.
Johns Hopkins University
Baltimore, Md.

Karin B. Nelson, M.D.
National Institute on Neurological
  Disorders and Stroke
Bethesda, Md.

Edward Oldfield, M.D., F.A.C.S.
National Institute on Neurological
  Disorders and Stroke
Bethesda, Md.

John W. Olney, M.D.
Washington University School of
  Medicine
St. Louis, Mo.

Herbert Pardes, M.D.
Columbia University College of
  Physicians and Surgeons
New York, N.Y.

Audrey S. Penn, M.D.
National Institute on Neurological
  Disorders and Stroke
Bethesda, Md.

Edward R. Perl, M.D.
University of North Carolina at
  Chapel Hill
Chapel Hill, N.C.

Michael E. Phelps, Ph.D.
UCLA School of Medicine
Los Angeles, Calif.

Jonathan H. Pincus, M.D.
Georgetown University School of
  Medicine
Washington, D.C.

Fred Plum, M.D.
Cornell University Medical College
New York, N.Y.

Michael I. Posner, Ph.D.
University of Oregon
Eugene, Oreg.

Robert M. Post, M.D.
National Institute of Mental Health
Bethesda, Md.

Donald L. Price, M.D.
Johns Hopkins University School of
  Medicine
Baltimore, Md.

Stanley B. Prusiner, M.D.
University of California, San
  Francisco
San Francisco, Calif.

Dominick P. Purpura, M.D.
Albert Einstein College of
  Medicine
Bronx, N.Y.

Dale Purves, M.D.
Duke University Medical Center
Durham, N.C.

Marcus E. Raichle, M.D.
Washington University School of
  Medicine
St. Louis, Mo.

Pasko Rakic, M.D., Ph.D.
Yale University School of
  Medicine
New Haven, Conn.

Judith L. Rapoport, M.D.
National Institute of Mental Health
Bethesda, Md.

Richard M. Restak, M.D.
George Washington University
  School of Medicine and Health
  Sciences
Washington, D.C.

James T. Robertson, M.D.
University of Tennessee,
  Memphis
Memphis, Tenn.

Robert G. Robinson, M.D.
University of Iowa College of
  Medicine
Iowa City, Iowa

Robert M. Rose, M.D.
The John D. and Catherine T.
  MacArthur Foundation
Chicago, Il.

Roger N. Rosenberg, M.D.
Southwestern Medical Center—
  University of Texas
Dallas, Tex.

Allen D. Roses, M.D.
Duke University Medical Center
Durham, N.C.

Lewis P. Rowland, M.D.
Columbia-Presbyterian Medical
  Center
New York, N.Y.

Gerald M. Rubin, Ph.D.
University of California,
  Berkeley
Berkeley, Calif.

Stephen J. Ryan, M.D.
University of Southern California
Los Angeles, Calif.

Murray B. Sachs, Ph.D.
Johns Hopkins University School of
  Medicine
Baltimore, Md.

Martin A. Samuels, M.D.
Brigham amd Women's Hospital
Boston, Mass.

Joshua R. Sanes, Ph.D.
Washington University School of
  Medicine
St. Louis, Mo.

Clifford B. Saper, M.D., Ph.D.
Harvard Medical School
Boston, Mass.

John L. Schwartz, M.D.
Psychiatric Times
Santa Ana, Calif.

Dennis J. Selkoe, M.D.
Brigham and Women's Hospital,
  Harvard Medical School
Boston, Mass.

Carla J. Shatz, Ph.D.
University of California, Berkeley
Berkeley, Calif.

Bennett A. Shaywitz, M.D.
Yale University School of Medicine
New Haven, Conn.

Sally E. Shaywitz, M.D.
Yale University School of Medicine
New Haven, Conn.

Eric M. Shooter, Ph.D.
Stanford University School of
  Medicine
Stanford, Calif.

Donald H. Silberberg, M.D.
Hospital of the University of
  Pennsylvania
Philadelphia, Pa.

Solomon H. Snyder, M.D.
Johns Hopkins University
Baltimore, Md.

Larry R Squire, Ph.D.
University of California, San Diego
San Diego, Calif.

Charles F. Stevens, M.D., Ph.D.
The Salk Institute for Biological
  Studies
La Jolla, Calif.

Paula Tallal, Ph.D.
Rutgers University at Newark
Newark, N.J.

Robert D. Terry, M.D.
University of California, San Diego
La Jolla, Calif.

Hans Thoenen, M.D.
Max-Planck Institute for Psychiatry
Martinsried, Germany

James F. Toole, M.D.
Bowman Gray School of Medicine
Winston-Salem, N.C.

Daniel C. Tosteson, M.D.
Harvard Medical School
Boston, Mass.

John Q. Trojanowski, M.D., Ph.D.
University of Pennsylvania School
  of Medicine
Philadelphia, Pa.

David C. Van Essen, Ph.D.
Washington University School of
  Medicine
St. Louis, Mo.

James D. Watson, Ph.D.
Cold Spring Harbor Laboratory
Cold Spring Harbor, N.Y.

Stanley J. Watson, M.D., Ph.D.
University of Michigan
Ann Arbor, Mich.

Stephen G. Waxman, M.D., Ph.D.
Yale University School of Medicine
New Haven, Conn.

Myrna Weissman, Ph.D.
Columbia University College of
  Physicians and Surgeons
New York, N.Y.

Nancy S. Wexler, Ph.D.
Columbia University
New York, N.Y.

Jack P. Whisnant, M.D.
Mayo Medical School
Rochester, Minn.

Torsten N. Wiesel, M.D.
The Rockefeller University
New York, N.Y.

Jan A. Witkowski, Ph.D.
Cold Spring Harbor Laboratory
Cold Spring Harbor, N.Y.

C. C. Wood, Ph.D.
Los Alamos National Laboratory
Los Alamos, N.M.

Robert H. Wurtz, Ph.D.
National Eye Institute
Bethesda, Md.

Richard Jed Wyatt, M.D.
National Institute of Mental Health
Washington, D.C.

Anne B. Young, M.D., Ph.D.
Massachusetts General Hospital
Boston, Mass.

Wise Young, M.D., Ph.D.
Bellevue Hospital
New York, N.Y.

Nicholas T. Zervas, M.D.
Massachusetts General Hospital
Boston, Mass.

Earl A. Zimmerman, M.D.
The Oregon Health Sciences
  University
Portland, Oreg.

BIBLIOGRAPHY

Aldwin, C. M., M. R. Levenson, A. Spiro III, and R. Bosse. "Does emotionality predict stress? Findings from the normative aging study." *J Pers Soc Psychol* 56, no. 4 (1989): 618–624.

Associated Press. "Vitamin E Found to Aid Immune System in Elderly." *Washington Post,* May 7, 1997, A22.

Baker, Beth. "'There's No Magic Bullet' Anti-Aging Humbug?" *AARP Bulletin,* April 1997.

Baltes, Paul B., and Margaret M. Baltes. *Successful Aging: Perspectives from the Behavioral Sciences.* New York: Cambridge University Press, 1990.

Barinaga, Marcia. "How Much Pain for Cardiac Gain?" *Science* 276 (1997): 1324–1327.

Bender, Kenneth J. "Vitamin E for Alzheimer's: Is Cautious Optimism Justified?" *Psychiatric Times,* June 1997, 28–29.

Bidlack, W. R. "Interrelationships of Food, Nutrition, Diet and Health: The National Association of State Universities and Land Grant Colleges White Paper." *J Am Coll Nutr* 15, no. 5 (1996): 422–433.

Booth, Wayne. *The Art of Growing Older: Writers on Living and Aging Selected with Personal Reflections.* Chicago: University of Chicago Press, 1992.

Borawski, E. A., J. M. Kinney, and E. Kahana. "The Meaning of Older Adults' Health Appraisals: Congruence with Health Status and Determinant of Mortality." *J Gerontol B Psychol Sci Soc Sci* 51, no. 3 (1996): S157–170.

Clements, Jonathan. "What to Do When Markets Run Wild? Stay Calm and Keep These Points in Mind." *Wall Street Journal,* August 19, 1997, C1.

Cobb, Stanley. "Presidential Address—1976. Social Support as a Moderator of Life Stress." *Psychosom Med* 38, no. 5 (1997): 300–314.

Cole, Thomas R., and Mary G. Winkler. *The Oxford Book of Aging: Reflections on the Journey of Life.* New York: Oxford University Press, 1994.

Colvin, Geoffrey. "How to Beat the Boomer Rush." *Fortune,* August 18, 1997, 59–63.

Crenshaw, Albert B. "Young People Need to Find Road to Financial Stability." *Washington Post,* March 2, 1997, H1, H8.

Eronen, Minna K. "Quality of Life Can Improve After Menopause." *J Am Giratr Soc* 45 (1997): 594–597.

Gerson, Michael J. "Do Do-gooders Do Much Good?" *U.S. News & World Report,* April 28, 1997.

Heilbrun, Carolyn G. *The Last Gift of Time: Life Beyond 60.* New York: Dial Press, 1997.

Horvitz, Leslie Alan. "Scientists and Shrinks Agree—Sad Hearts Tempt Grim Reaper." *Insight,* July 7–14, 1997, 38–39.

Jazwinski, S. Michal. "Longevity, Genes, and Aging." *Science* 273 (1996): 54–58.

Kaku, Michio. *Visions: How Science Will Revolutionize the 21st Century.* New York: Doubleday, Anchor Books, 1997.

Kawas, Claudia. "Estrogen Replacement May Halve Risk of Alzheimer's Disease." *Neurology* 48 (1997): 1517–1521.

Khachaturian, Zaven S. "Can New Findings About Alzheimer's Disease Stop Its Theft of Mind and Spirit?" *The Sciences,* July–August 1997, 21–25.

Kitcher, Philip. "Whose Self Is It, Anyway?" *The Sciences,* September–October 1997, 58–62.

Krucoff, Carol. "Can't Get to the Gym? Activate Your Life." *Washington Post,* April 8, 1997, 20.

———. "Weightlifting for Weight Loss." *Washington Post,* October 29, 1996, 20.

Levy, B. "Improving Memory in Old Age Through Implicit Self-Stereotyping." *J Pers Soc Psychol* 71, no. 6 (1996): 1092–1107.

Lindgren, A. M., K. Svardsudd, and G. Tibblin. "Factors Related to Perceived Health Among Elderly People: The Albertina Project." *Age and Ageing* 23, no. 4 (1994): 328–333.

Loeb, Marshall. *Marshall Loeb's Lifetime Financial Strategies: Your Ultimate Guide to Future Wealth and Security.* Boston: Little, Brown and Co., 1996.

Mann, Denise. *Moderate Exercise Promotes Longevity.* Medical Tribune News Service, 1996.

Marx, Jean. "Searching for Drugs That Combat Alzheimer's." *Science* 273 (1996): 50–53.

McCrae, R. R. "Age Differences in the Use of Coping Mechanisms." *J Gerontol* 37, no. 4 (1982): 454–460.

Miller, Richard A. "The Aging Immune System: Primer and Prospectus." *Science* 273 (1996): 70–73.

Murray, Christopher J. L., and Alan D. Lopez. "Gender Gap in Life Expenctancy Will Widen: Tobacco Use Major Cause." *Lancet* 349 (1997): 1498–1504.

Nishisaka, S., K. Utoguchi, T. Mizoue, N. Tokui, I. Ogimoto, M. Ikeda, and T. Yoshimura. "The Association of Self-Rated Health and Mortality—a Seven-Year Follow-up Study of a Japanese Community." *Sangyo Ika Daigaku Zasshi* 18, no. 2 (1996): 119–131.

Perls, Thomas T. "The Oldest Old." *Scientific American,* January 1995, 70–75.

Perna, F. M., N. Schneiderman, and A. LaPerriere. "Psychological Stress, Exercise and Immunity." *Int J Sports Med* 18, suppl. 1 (1997): S78–83.

"Pharmacology of Aging Processes: Methods of Assessment and Potential Interventions." In *Annals of the New York Academy of Sciences* 717, ed. Imre Zs.-Nagy, Denham Harman, and Kenichi Kitani. New York: New York Academy of Sciences, 1994.

Poon, Leonard W., Martha H. Bramlett, Philip A. Holtsberg, Mary Ann Johnson, and Peter Martin. "Who Will Survive to 105?" In *1997 Medical and Health Annual*. Chicago: Encyclopaedia Britannica, 1997.

Reiman, Eric M., M.D., Richard D. Lane, M.D., Geoffrey L. Ahern, M.D., Ph.D., Gary E. Schwartz, Ph.D., Richard J. Davidson, Ph.D., Karl J. Friston, M.B.B.S., Yun Lang-sheng, Ph.D., and Chen Kewei, Ph.D. "Neuro-anatomical Correlates of Externally and Internally Generated Human Emotion." *Am J Psychiatry* 154 (1997): 918–925.

Roush, Wade. "Live Long and Prosper?" *Science* 273 (1996): 42–46.

Samuelson, Robert J. "R.I.P., Early Retirement?" *Newsweek*, November 17, 1997, 61.

Sapolsky, Robert M. *Why Zebras Don't Get Ulcers: A Guide to Stress, Stress-Related Diseases and Coping*. New York: W. H. Freeman, 1994.

Shepard, R. J., and P. N. Sheck. "Impact of Physical Activity and Sport on the Immune System." *Rev Environ Health* 11, no. 3 (1996): 133–147.

Sohal, Rajindar S., and Richard Weindruch. "Oxidative Stress, Caloric Restriction, and Aging." *Science* 273 (1996): 59–63.

Stanley, Thomas. "How to Become a Millionaire: Very Practical Lessons from Those Who Really Made It." *Bottom Line* 18, no. 9 (May 1, 1997): 1–3.

———. "$1 Million Worth of Secrets." *U.S. News & World Report*, June 9, 1997, 90–92.

Steptoe, A., J. Wardle, T. M. Pollard, L. Canaan, and G. J. Davies. "Stress, Social Support and Health-Related Behavior: A Study of Smoking, Alcohol Consumption and Physical Exercise." *J Psychosom Res* 41, no. 2 (1996): 171–180.

Susman, Ed. "Vitamin E Supplementation May Delay Progression of Alzheimer's Disease." *Medical Tribune*, May 22, 1997.

Wall, Ginita, and Victoria F. Collins. *Your Next Fifty Years: A Completely New Way to Look at How, When and If You Should Retire*. New York: Henry Holt, 1997.

Wickelgren, Ingrid. "Estrogen Stakes Claim to Cognition." *Science* 276 (1997): 675–678.

———. "For the Cortex, Neuron Loss May Be Less Than Thought." *Science* 273 (1996): 48–50.

Williams, Redford B. "Job Stress Linked to Health-Damaging Psychosocial Factors in Women." *Arch Gen Psychiatry* 54 (1997): 543–548.

INDEX

neurotransmitters *(continued)*
  brain functioning and, 43, 205
  depression and, 28, 170–71, 172
  strokes and, 108–9
New England Centenarian Study, 13
Nixon, Richard, 62
norepinephrine, 171
Norstrom, Jane, 185
Norton Simon, Inc., 125–26
nostalgia, 117–18, 119
nursing homes, 120–21, 169
nutrition. *See* diet and nutrition

obesity, 184 (*see also* weight control)
optimism, 13, 26, 72–81
osteoporosis, 185
Outward Bound, 58

Paige, Satchel, 187
pain treatment, 128–29
panic attacks, 130
parasympathetic nervous system, 59, 60

Parkinson's disease, 32, 36, 44, 128, 210, 211, 217
pensions, 136–37
Perls, Thomas T., 13, 207
personality, 10, 12–13, 46–47, 82–86, 149–50
pessimism, 74–77, 81
pet ownership, 84
PET scanning, 33–34, 218, 220
Phelps, Mike, 33–34
Phoenix House, 148
phosphorus, 191
physical exams, 112
physical fitness. *See* exercise
Poon, Leonard, 11–12, 13, 67
positron emission tomography (PET), 33–34, 218, 220
Powell, Colin, 146
practical wisdom, 41
predictability, stress and, 61–62
problem-finding perspective, 156
problem-solving skills, 95
Prochaska, James, 197
programmed senescence, 10–11, 200